Telecourse Guide for

LIVING ◆ WITH Health

Fourth Edition

Donna Beck Richards, R.N., M.S.

Produced by:

DALLAS

DALLAS TeleLearning
Dallas County Community College District

THOMSON
WADSWORTH

Australia • Canada • Mexico • Singapore • Spain
United Kingdon • United States

The Telecourse Guide for Living with Health is produced by the Dallas County Community College District, DALLAS TeleLearning, in association with the Wadsworth Group.

1 2 3 4 5 6 7 05 04 03 02

For more information contact
Wadsworth/Thomson Learning
10 Davis Drive
Belmont, CA 94002-3098
USA

For more information about our products, contact us:
Thomson Learning Academic Resource Center
1-800-423-0563
http://www.wadsworth.com

International Headquarters
Thomson Learning
International Division
290 Harbor Drive, 2nd Floor
Stamford, CT 06902-7477
USA

Asia
Thomson Learning
60 Albert Complex, #15-01
Singapore 189969

UK/Europe/Middle East/South Africa
Thomson Learning
Berkshire House
168-173 High Holborn
London WC1V 7AA
United Kingdom

Canada
Nelson Thomson Learning
1120 Birchmount Road
Toronto, Ontario M1K 5G4
Canada

Richard Bach, *Jonathan Livingston Seagull*, New York, Macmillan, 1990.
Rahima Baldwin and Terra Palmarini, *Pregnant Feelings*, Berkeley, Calif., Celestial Arts, 1986.
Norman Cousins, *Anatomy of an Illness as Perceived by the Patient: Reflections on Healing and Regeneration*, New York, Bantam, 1981.
Larry Dossey, M.D., *Beyond Illness*, New York, Random House, 1985.
Robert A. Johnson, *We*, San Francisco, Harper, 1985.
Elisabeth Kübler-Ross, M.D., *On Life After Death*, Berkeley, Calif., Celestial Arts Publisher, 1991.
Anne Morrow Lindbergh, *Gift from the Sea*, New York, Pantheon Books, 1975.

ISBN 0-534-58306-7

Without the high and the low, the hot and the cold, life would be a seamless, undifferentiated experience of sameness. Without the rhythms of health and illness and birth and death, we would fall heir not to a state of pristine perfection, but to one of experiential anesthesia. Our health strategy must always be supplemented with this awareness. For if we ever achieved our goal of total health, we would find, not fulfillment, but emptiness. Health, if seen as wholeness, guards against this dreadful error, for the whole contains all—even we must all recall, the opposites of birth and death, pain and pleasure, illness and health.

—Larry Dossey, M.D.
Beyond Illness

No project such as this is ever the work of one person. Many people shared the commitment to *Living with Health* and I thank each of them.

To Paul Bosner, Director of Production, who also functioned as one of the producers, I owe thanks for an incredible experience, for keeping us on track, and for sharing a lifetime of experience with this neophyte. Thanks to Mark Birnbaum, Producer/Director, for his creativity and sensitivity to the subject matter and putting up with the content specialist. To Nora Coto Busby, Instructional Designer, I owe the instructional quality of this course, and thanks for being a real friend who kept me centered throughout. Karen C. Austen, Researcher, did well-focused research, too many other duties to mention, and asked questions that made us all think. David Molina, Associate Producer, kept us all organized and on the road, and had the answer to any question we could ever think of.

Without the work of Darise Error and Michelle Miller, Production Assistants, there would have been no video programs. I thank Letitia Richardson and Lannie Waggy for all those details that added to the project. My admiration goes to Janet Fulton, Vicki Metz, and Michael Coleman for their talented editing of the video and to the camera and audio experts who brought the whole thing to life. Thanks to Betsy Turner and Evelyn Wong for their most competent work and untiring commitment to the quality of this edition. Other special people to this project were Pamela K. Quinn, Assistant Chancellor/LeCroy Center, and all the staff at the Center who were so involved. Thanks also to Margot Olson, Test Design Specialist, and Nancy Ward of The Word Works. Appreciation to all those on the advisory committees who shared their wisdom to improve my efforts. Finally, thanks to all those special people who shared their lives with us, and all you students who taught me so much through the years.

For the fourth edition, thanks to Karen Austen for her careful work in keying the pages of this guide to the tenth edition of the textbook and to Evelyn Wong for her skillful work in bringing the pieces together once again.

—Donna Beck Richards, R.N., M.S.

Contents

To You, the Student

Welcome to Living with Health! You and I are about to take a long journey. We will travel over 30,000 miles, meet some of the nation's top experts in the fields of medicine and health, and share the lives of dozens of special people. If I just described these people to you, you might wonder why I define them as "special," because they are much like you and me—just "folks" living their lives, coping with the ups and downs that life has to offer. You will find as you meet them, that indeed they are special, as are you and I. Each of us is unique, yet we all share some of the same ups and downs, hopes and fears, pain and celebration.

As we travel and visit with these people, we will see their lifestyles, hear about their experiences, and understand what it takes to achieve and maintain a high quality of health and well-being. Throughout our travels in this course, we will be looking at health in its dimensions: physical, emotional, intellectual, social, environmental, and spiritual. All these aspects of our being come together to make us a whole, healthy person. In our time together, we will discuss many of the topics related to health within this framework of the dimensions of health. We will discover that health is a dynamic process rather than a static point. We will find that most of our good health is within our control and is our responsibility to maintain.

The fifteen months that I have committed to the development of *Living with Health* have been life-changing for me. I hope the months that we spend together will change yours as well. The purpose of *Living with Health* is to give you tools to make lifestyle choices and decisions that will improve the quality of your health and well-being. Whether you choose them to shape your own life will, of course, be your decision. I very much hope you will find these tools useful to your life.

—Donna Beck Richards, R.N., M.S.

Telecourse Organization

Living with Health is designed as a comprehensive learning system consisting of three elements: telecourse guide, textbook, and video programs.

TELECOURSE GUIDE

The telecourse guide for this course is:

Richards, Donna Beck. *Telecourse Guide for Living with Health,* 4th ed. Belmont, CA: Wadsworth Thomson Learning , 2003.

This telecourse guide acts as your daily instructor. For each lesson it gives you a lesson assignment, an overview, learning objectives, key terms, text and video focus points, individual health plans, related activities, and a practice test. If you follow the telecourse guide recommendations and view each lesson carefully, you should successfully accomplish all of the requirements for this course.

TEXTBOOK

In addition to the telecourse guide, the textbook required for this course is:

Hales, Dianne. *An Invitation to Health,* 10th ed. Belmont, CA: Wadsworth Thomson Learning Publishing Company, 2002.

VIDEO PROGRAMS

The video program series for this course is:

Living with Health

Each video program is correlated to a specific reading assignment for that lesson. The video programs are packed with information, so watch them closely.

If the lessons are broadcast more than once in your area, or if video or audio tapes are available at your college, you might find it helpful to watch the video programs again or listen to audio tapes for review. Since examination questions will be taken from the video programs as well as from the textbook, careful attention to both is vital to your success.

TELECOURSE PLUS

An online interactive option is available to students whose institutions have opted to license it. The web activities are useful for working with "real-time" information related to the lesson content and objectives. If your course includes this PLUS component, please consult your instructor for the course website address and required password.

Telecourse Guidelines

Follow these guidelines as you study the material presented in each lesson:

1. LESSON ASSIGNMENT—
   Review the Lesson Assignment in order to schedule your time appropriately. Pay careful attention; the titles and numbers of the textbook chapter, the telecourse guide lesson, and the video program may be different from one another.

2. OVERVIEW—
   Read the Overview for an introduction to the lesson material.

3. LEARNING OBJECTIVES—
   Review the Learning Objectives and pay particular attention to the lesson material that relates to them.

4. KEY TERMS—
   Look for these items as you proceed through the lesson assignments. Be able to discuss them upon completion of this lesson.

5. TEXT FOCUS POINTS—
   To get the most from your reading, review the Text Focus Points, then read the assignment. You may want to write responses or notes to reinforce what you have learned.

6. VIDEO FOCUS POINTS—
   To get the most from the video segment of the lesson, review the Video Focus Points, then watch the video. You may want to write responses or notes to reinforce what you have learned.

7. INDIVIDUAL HEALTH PLAN—
   This portion of the lesson is designed to enable you to use the information you have learned in your own life situation to improve the quality of your life. You should do any exercise assigned, complete the journal portion of the plan, then put this portion of the health plan into practice in your life.

8. RELATED ACTIVITIES—
   These activities are not required unless your instructor assigns them. They are offered as suggestions to help you learn more about the material presented in this lesson.

9. PRACTICE TEST—
   After reading the assignment and watching the video, you should be able to answer the Practice Test questions. Tests also include essay questions that are similar to the Text Focus Points and the Video Focus Points. When you have completed the Practice Test questions, turn to the Answer Key to score your answers.

10. ANSWER KEY—
    Use the Answer Key at the end of the lesson to check your answers or to locate material related to each question of the Practice Test.

Lesson 1

Invitation to Health

If you can force your heart and nerve and sinew
To serve your turn long after they are gone,
And so hold on when there is nothing in you
Except the Will which says to them: "Hold on"

—Rudyard Kipling

LESSON ASSIGNMENT

Review the following assignment in order to schedule your time appropriately. Pay careful attention; the titles and numbers of the textbook chapter, the telecourse guide lesson, and the video program may be different from one another.

Text:

Hales, *An Invitation to Health,*
Chapter 1, "An Invitation to Health for the Twenty-First Century," pp. 12–37.

Video:

"Invitation to Health"
from the series *Living with Health.*

OVERVIEW

How do you define health? If you think merely in terms of getting exercise and eating the "right" foods, you are missing more than four-fifths of the ingredients of health. If you define health as the absence of disease, you are missing even more.

Come with us into a much more exciting and interesting world of health and wellness. Think of the dimensions that define our health—physical, psychological/emotional, intellectual, spiritual, and social. The environmental dimension is often included since environmental forces impact our health in a significant way. Each of these interact and interrelate to form who and what we are. Each has a major impact on our well-being. If all are not nurtured and maintained, we will be less than whole.

A significant part of our being will be needy. In each of us, one or another of these dimensions may be more or less developed, but they are there.

To add to the complexity and wonder of all this, our lifestyle and its components are the most important influences on these dimensions of health. So how we live our lives has more to do with our health than any other component. Before we talk more about the components of lifestyle today, think for a moment about how our lifestyles have changed through the generations. Our lifestyle has evolved from that of hunting and gathering food to one of sedentary work and fast food establishments. At the same time, strides in medicine and technology have conquered many of the diseases that killed our ancestors. Until recently, our health was considered more a matter of luck than individual responsibility.

Many bacterial and viral diseases have been conquered that were out of our own control to prevent. We now realize that the killer diseases of today frequently are related intimately to lifestyle. In other words, our lifestyle may be killing us. If the idea of killing yourself is startling, let's talk more about what we mean by the lifestyles that have such positive and negative influence on our health.

Our lifestyle means the way we spend the major parts of our lives: working, communicating, recreating, relating, consuming, etc. How we design and structure these components determines, to a large degree, how healthy we are. Though we cannot change our heredity, we do have the power to make the lifestyle decisions that will improve the quality of our health.

Making these decisions, setting our goals, assessing our health status, and then actually carrying out our plan is not always easy. We have to constantly evaluate our progress, sometimes adjust our goals, and just "keep on trucking." The outcome is definitely worth the effort, for there is no doubt that we will improve the quality of our lives—**and have lots of fun while we are doing it!**

LEARNING OBJECTIVES

Goal

You should be able to explain the dimensions of health, the principles of health promotion, the impact of lifestyle on health, and the importance of health goals.

Objectives

Upon completion of this lesson, you should be able to:

1. Define health in terms of the integration and balance of the dimensions of health.
2. Explain the principles and goals of prevention, and differentiate prevention from protection.
3. Discuss the relationships of culture, economics, health care, lifestyle choices, self-efficacy, and other factors on one's health behavior.
4. Explain the importance of health goals and the principles of health promotion and create a plan to change or create a health behavior.
5. Describe the Healthy People 2000 and Healthy People 2010 initiatives.

KEY TERMS

Look for these items as you proceed through the lesson assignments. Be able to discuss them upon completion of this lesson.

health
wellness
health promotion
self-efficacy
locus of control
self-talk
prevention
protection
genes
promotion

TEXT FOCUS POINTS

The following focus points are designed to help you get the most from the text. Review them, then read the assignment. You may want to write notes to reinforce what you have learned.

Text: Hales, *An Invitation to Health,* Chapter 1, pp. 12–37.

1. Identify and explain the dimensions of health and how they relate to total wellness.

2. Discuss the relationship between world/culture, economics, and health care.

3. Describe some health challenges to ethnically diverse and "underserved" groups in the United States. What is the importance of the Healthy People 2000 and Healthy People 2010 initiatives?

4. What influences must you understand in order to understand health behavior?

5. What steps are involved in setting goals and making decisions that have immediate and long-term effects on your health?

6. How do self-efficacy, locus of control, reinforcement, and self-talk influence your success in changing health behavior?

7. Explain the principles and goals of prevention, and differentiate prevention from protection.

8. Why are genes and genetic research important in health?

9. Explain the principles of health promotion.

VIDEO FOCUS POINTS

The following focus points are designed to help you get the most from the video segment of this lesson. Review them, then watch the video. You may want to write notes to reinforce what you have learned.

Video: "Invitation to Health"

1. How are definitions of health and wellness different today than in the past?

2. Why is it important that the dimensions, which include physical, emotional, intellectual, social, and spiritual, be balanced in one's life?

3. Explain the importance of lifestyle decisions on one's health and the balance of the dimensions. Include differences from person to person and from time to time.

INDIVIDUAL HEALTH PLAN

This portion of the lesson is designed to enable you to use the information you have learned in your own life situation to improve the quality of your life. You should do any exercise assigned, complete the journal portion of the plan, then put this portion of the health plan into practice in your life.

> Complete the "Wellness Inventory" on pp. 1–9 of your textbook. Once you have completed it, begin your journal writing by developing a written plan to improve your health. Include your health and wellness goals in this exercise.

RELATED ACTIVITIES

These activities are not required unless your instructor assigns them. They are offered as suggestions to help you learn more about the material presented in this lesson.

1. Conduct interviews with some of your friends and family. Evaluate their lifestyle choices, based on what you have learned from this lesson.

2. If you smoke, stop! (Additional information may be found in Lesson 19.)

3. After consulting with your instructor and possibly your physician, begin an exercise program. (Refer to Lesson 5 for additional information.)

PRACTICE TEST

After reading the assignment and watching the video, you should be able to answer the Practice Test questions. Tests also include essay questions that are similar to the Text Focus Points and the Video Focus Points. When you have completed the Practice Test questions, turn to the Answer Key to score your answers.

Multiple-Choice

Select the one choice that best answers the question.

1. Which of the following best describes "wellness"?
   A. Absence of disease or infirmity
   B. Striving to achieve optimal health
   C. Being socially healthy
   D. Recovering from illness

2. The concept of "underserved" groups in health care refers to __________.
   A. people who are from minority groups
   B. homeless Americans
   C. women
   D. all of the above

3. Which of the following seems to be the primary factor in decreasing a person's risk factor for disease?
   A. Money
   B. Prestige
   C. Education
   D. Stamina

4. Predisposing factors related to health behaviors are __________.
   A. pre-existing factors such as culture, belief, and values
   B. only products of genetic make-up
   C. learned skills, accessible facilities, and physical capacities
   D. derived from praise from significant others

5. Which model in changing health behaviors involves rewarding yourself when you make positive changes?
   A. Moral
   B. Enlightenment
   C. Behavioral
   D. Medical

6. Immunizing a child against polio would be an example of __________.
   A. primary prevention
   B. consumer education
   C. secondary prevention
   D. health treatment

7. All of the following might be key factors to consider in assessing risks relative to certain behaviors EXCEPT __________.
   A. possible benefits that outweigh risks.
   B. alternative behaviors to the risk.
   C. the framing of the risk.
   D. whether genetic testing will eliminate the risk.

8. All of the following might be examples of health promotion programs EXCEPT __________.
   A. the local drugstore conducts a cholesterol screening
   B. Students against Destructive Decisions (SADD) gives a free lecture
   C. someone goes to the doctor when they are sick
   D. Weight Watchers offers a free introductory program

9. Health is defined as __________.
   A. being free of disease
   B. feeling happy
   C. functioning at a high level
   D. staying alive

10. When the dimensions of health are out of balance, the individual is most likely to feel __________.
    A. disease free
    B. ill at ease
    C. stress free
    D. in control

11. Most major health problems of today are attributed to __________.
    A. infection
    B. lifestyle
    C. immune system problems
    D. viruses

Fill-in-the-Blank

Insert the correct word or words in the blank for each item.

12. Being happily married would be an example of the component of __________ health.

13. Praise from family and friends, rewards from teachers or parents, or encouragement and recognition are examples of ___________ factors that influence health behaviors.

14. Psychologist Albert Bandurra found that individuals with _______ _________ who believed that they could succeed with change actually succeeded.

15. Quality of life, resulting in a high level of functioning in all aspects of living, is a definition for ___________.

16. One of the major keys to good health is our choice of _________________.

True-False

If the statement is true, write "T" to the left of the statement. If the statement (or any part of the statement) is false, write "F" to the left of the statement.

17. Wellness is a generic term that refers to a healthful approach to living.

18. One can live a very healthy life even if one or two of the dimensions are out of balance.

ANSWER KEY

The following provides the answers and references for the Practice Test questions. Focus Points are referenced using the following abbreviations:

T = Text and V = Video

	Answers	Learning Objectives	Focus Points	References
1.	B	1	T1	Hales, p. 14
2.	D	3	T3	Hales, p. 21
3.	C	3	T2	Hales, p. 25
4.	A	3	T4	Hales, pp. 26
5.	C	3	T5	Hales, p. 28
6.	A	4	T7	Hales, p. 30
7.	D	4	T8	Hales, p. 31
8.	C	4	T9	Hales, p. 31
9.	C	1	V1	Video
10.	B	1	V2	Video
11.	B	3	V3	Video
12.	social	1	T1	Hales, p. 17
13.	reinforcing	3	T4	Hales, p. 27
14.	self-efficacy	3	T6	Hales, p. 28
15.	health	1	V1	Video
16.	lifestyle	3	V3	Video
17.	T	1	V1	Video
18.	F	1	V2	Video

Lesson 2

Stress

Dig the well before you are thirsty.

—Chinese proverb

LESSON ASSIGNMENT

Review the following assignment in order to schedule your time appropriately. Pay careful attention; the titles and numbers of the textbook chapter, the telecourse guide lesson, and the video program may be different from one another.

Text:

Hales, *An Invitation to Health,*
Chapter 2, "Personal Stress Management," pp. 38–65.

Video:

"Stress"
from the series *Living with Health.*

OVERVIEW

When asked whether stress is good or bad, most of us will say **bad** without hesitation. The fact is, if you do not have stress in your life, you are **dead**! Stress actually keeps us alive! In reality stress is neither good nor bad, yet it is both good and bad. Now are you thoroughly confused? The way in which we cope with stress is the factor that makes each stress a positive or negative factor in our lives.

We all encounter stress every day in our lives, some tiny and routine, some large, unavoidable, and terrifying, and some very intense and personal in our relationships with others. Our ability to understand the nature of stress, our physiological and psychological responses to stress, and how we manage and reduce the negative effects of stress have major impact on our health and well-being.

No matter what the stress is, if we perceive a threat, our bodies have certain physical ways of responding. Increased heart rate, rapid breathing, elevated blood pressure, and increased mental alertness are all part of a three-stage process, defined by Dr. Hans Selye, as the general adaptation syndrome (GAS). The brain, autonomic nervous system, and endocrine system are all involved in our complex physiological response to stress.

Our personality also has a great deal to do with how well we cope with stress. If we believe in ourselves and our abilities, view stress as a normal part of life, and look at life changes in a positive way, we will be far more likely to cope effectively with the stress in our lives.

Stress, however, can have a very negative effect on our behavior and our ability to resist or withstand various diseases. If we are not coping with stress effectively, we may turn to drugs, alcohol, or tobacco instead of dealing with the stress. We may also become depressed, lack concentration, and even engage in acts that increase our risk of injury. Stress has also been linked to an increased risk of many diseases such as hypertension, heart disease, diabetes, peptic ulcers, mental disorders, and others. Burnout and other job-related stress can also present major problems in our lives.

Stress is an inevitable part of our lives and in fact can be a very positive force in our health. Our goal should not be to remove stress from our lives but to manage it and reduce its negative effects. We can use stress to motivate us to achieve a higher quality of life.

Simple "band-aid" stress management techniques, such as taking a break from working or studying, surprisingly can offer immediate relief. More complex techniques, such as progressive relaxation, meditation, and biofeedback training, are relatively easy to learn and can make a real difference in our lives. In addition to these, learning to approach our lives and stressors in different ways, managing our time effectively, practicing general good health measures, and believing in ourselves and our abilities will give us the tools we need to manage our stress in a healthy way.

LEARNING OBJECTIVES

Goal

You should be able to explain stress, its physiological and psychological effects, the impact of stress on the individual, and the most common stress management techniques.

Objectives

Upon completion of this lesson, the student should be able to:

1. Explain stress, its relationship to health, the general adaptation syndrome, and techniques and coping strategies for managing stress.

2. List types of personal, social, and other stressors and explain how these can cause stress.

3. Describe the symptoms of stress-related adjustment disorders and the relationship of stress to heart disease, high blood pressure, the immune system, and digestive disorders.

KEY TERMS

Look for these items as you proceed through the lesson assignments. Be able to discuss them upon completion of this lesson.

stress
stressor
eustress
distress
general adaption syndrome (GAS)
psychoneuroimmunology
homeostasis
adaptive response
allostasis
burnout
coping mechanisms
progressive relaxation
visualization
guided imagery
meditation
mindfulness
biofeedback
adjustment disorder
posttraumatic stress disorder (PTSD)
migraine headache

TEXT FOCUS POINTS

The following focus points are designed to help you get the most from the text. Review them, then read the assignment. You may want to write notes to reinforce what you have learned.

Text: Hales, *An Invitation to Health*, Chapter 2, pp. 38–65.

1. Define stress and stressors, and use the general adaptation syndrome to explain how stress relates to health.
2. List some personal causes of stress and discuss how their effects can be prevented or minimized.
3. What are the major social stressors? How can these cause stress?
4. Discuss some of the techniques that are helpful in managing stress.
5. Describe the symptoms of posttraumatic stress syndrome.
6. Explain the relationship of stress to heart disease, high blood pressure, the immune system, and digestive disorders and how you can improve your resistance to stress.

VIDEO FOCUS POINTS

The following focus points are designed to help you get the most from the video segment of this lesson. Review them, then watch the video. You may want to write notes to reinforce what you have learned.

Video: "Stress"

1. Explain and give examples of cataclysmic, personal, and background stressors.
2. What are situational stressors normally defined by the dimensions of health and how can they affect the individual?
3. Describe the body's physiologic response to stress.
4. Discuss several healthy ways to manage and cope with stress.

INDIVIDUAL HEALTH PLAN

This portion of the lesson is designed to enable you to use the information you have learned in your own life situation to improve the quality of your life. You should do any exercise assigned, complete the journal portion of the plan, then put this portion of the health plan into practice in your life.

> Using the Self-Survey "Student Stress Scale" on page 47, determine your level of stress. (On question 16 of the survey, substitute spouse for girlfriend or boyfriend if you are married.) In your journal, describe those aspects of your life that you would most like to change. Develop some plans based on the information in this lesson, and write out these plans. Begin working on your plan with the part of the plan you wish, then move to the next part. Don't try to do everything at once.

RELATED ACTIVITIES

These activities are not required unless your instructor assigns them. They are offered as suggestions to help you learn more about the material presented in this lesson.

> Learn and practice one of the relaxation or other techniques for managing stress.

PRACTICE TEST

After reading the assignment and watching the video, you should be able to answer the Practice Test questions. Tests also include essay questions that are similar to the Text Focus Points and the Video Focus Points. When you have completed the Practice Test questions, turn to the Answer Key to score your answers.

Multiple-Choice

Select the one choice that best answers the question.

1. The nonspecific responses of the body to any demand made upon it is a definition of __________.
   A. homeostasis
   B. stress
   C. excitement
   D. stressors

2. During which stage of the general adaptation syndrome does the body focus internal resources to maintain balance?
   A. Adaptation
   B. Alarm
   C. Resistance
   D. Exhaustion

3. The fact that exposure to stress may not cause disease symptoms for a long time supports the concept that __________.
   A. responses to stressors vary
   B. stress has little impact on physical health
   C. stress effects are cumulative
   D. stress affects people in different ways

4. Students most susceptible to exam stress tend to be those who __________.
   A. believe they will do poorly
   B. see tests as extremely threatening
   C. are preoccupied with failing
   D. all of the above

5. Which of the following is the leading killer of young people in inner-city communities in the United States?
   A. Drug abuse
   B. Accidental poisoning
   C. Murder
   D. Suicide

6. You consistently put off studying for exams until the last minute, you never complete one assignment before starting another, and you rarely turn in papers on time. You are experiencing __________.
   A. procrastination
   B. poor time management
   C. type B behaviors
   D. eustress

7. A key sign of postraumatic stress syndrome (disorder) in an individual is __________.
   A. a general increase in distress
   B. a general increase in distress and eustress.
   C. eustress and impairment
   D. coping and impairment

8. All of the following may be stress-related disorders that you could experience as a result of constant exposure to stressors EXCEPT __________.
   A. breaking out with acne during finals week
   B. unexplained chronic diarrhea
   C. getting an upset stomach when eating spicy food
   D. experiencing a bout with asthma only when pressured

9. Traffic delays and a busy job are examples of __________.
   A. cataclysmic stress
   B. personal stress
   C. background stress
   D. spiritual stress

10. Sustained levels of stress, over the long term, have __________.
    A. possible effects on immune function
    B. proven effect on lifestyles
    C. only effect on emotional health
    D. little effect on physiological function

11. An individual can cope with stresses by allocating some time for relaxation while __________.
    A. eliminating all problems at once
    B. solving one problem at a time
    C. ignoring all problems
    D. trying to stay busier

Fill-in-the-Blank

Insert the correct word or words in the blank for each item.

12. __________ are the things that upset or excite us and force the body to react.

13. _______ is a state of physical, emotional, and mental exhaustion brought on by repeated emotional pressure.

14. The relaxation technique that involves creating mental pictures that calm and focus the mind is known as guided imagery or ____________.

15. Stressors frequently related to communication problems are __________ stressors.

16. The body adjusts itself to respond to stressors in the _________ stage.

True-False

If the statement is true, write "T" to the left of the statement. If the statement (or any part of the statement) is false, write "F" to the left of the statement.

17. Personal stressors are intense, powerful situations that affect the individual rather than large groups.

18. The body's physiological response to stress is quite unpredictable and varies from individual to individual.

ANSWER KEY

The following provides the answers and references for the Practice Test questions. Focus Points are referenced using the following abbreviations:
T = Text and V = Video

	Answers	Learning Objectives	Focus Points	References
1.	B	1	T1	Hales, p. 40
2.	C	1	T1	Hales, p. 40
3.	C	2	T2	Hales, p. 43
4.	D	2	T2	Hales, p. 48
5.	C	2	T3	Hales, p. 54
6.	B	1	T4	Hales, p. 58
7.	A	3	T5	Hales, p. 60
8.	C	3	T6	Hales, p. 60
9.	C	2	V1	Video
10.	A	1	V3	Video
11.	B	1	V4	Video
12.	Stressors	1	T1	Hales, p. 40
13.	Burnout	2	T2	Hales, p. 52
14.	visualization	1	T4	Hales, p. 57
15.	social	2	V2	Video
16.	alarm	1	V3	Video
17.	T	2	V1	Video
18.	F	1	V3	Video

Lesson 3

Emotional Health

Simplification of outward life is not enough. It is merely the outside. But I am starting with the outside. I am looking at the outside of a shell, the outside of my life—the shell. The complete answer is not to be found on the outside, in an outward mode of living. This is only a technique, a road to grace. The final answer, I know, is always inside. But the outside can give a clue, can help one find the inward answer. One is free, like the hermit crab, to change one's shell.

—Anne Morrow Lindbergh, *Gift from the Sea*

LESSON ASSIGNMENT

Review the following assignment in order to schedule your time appropriately. Pay careful attention; the titles and numbers of the textbook chapter, the telecourse guide lesson, and the video program may be different from one another.

Text:

Hales, *An Invitation to Health,*
Chapter 3, "Psychological Health," pp. 66–70, pp. 72–92, and pp. 98–102.
It will be helpful if you read completely through the chapter before beginning on this lesson.

Video:

"Emotional Health"
from the series *Living with Health.*

OVERVIEW

When we think of a "healthy" person, we often think first of the physical dimension of health. In reality, our psychological health is probably a much more important indicator of our overall health. Psychological health encompasses the two states of our minds: the emotional or feeling part, and the mental or thinking, intellectual part. Our mind lets us feel the range of emotions: love, joy, pleasure, anger, and sadness. If we feel emotionally healthy, we feel better physically and can cope with physical illness. Our minds define who we are, set our goals, and determine what we will become and how happy and satisfying our lives will be.

Our emotions even have strong physical effects on our bodies. Heart rate, blood volume, blood pressure, electrodermal responses, muscle potential, and brain wave patterns all respond to our emotional states. It is interesting that even though we all experience these physical changes and label them as emotions, we differ in how we define a particular emotion. One person may feel afraid, while another experiencing the same physical changes may feel anger. Again, these examples of our individual differences reflect the ways we learned—by association and by observation.

We all wish our lives would be filled with nothing but positive, happy emotions. In reality, we must frequently deal with negative emotions, conflict, and stress. Anger and anxiety are normal emotions, and most of us have to deal with minor depression occasionally. When we experience these "down" times it is important to remember that there are effective ways to deal with them and turn the negative into a positive. We often use defense mechanisms. These mental strategies protect us from the anxiety associated with painful emotions. We use defense mechanisms to avoid dealing with the painful emotion or problem itself. We may rationalize or deny reality to avoid facing the issue. Some of this is perfectly normal. The trouble comes when we use these too frequently instead of coping with our problems.

Many of us and many of our loved ones will experience emotional disorders at some time. It is important to know that mental health and mental illness are on a continuum with many shadings between extremes. Most emotional problems, like most physical problems, respond well to treatment. Unfortunately, people sometimes are hesitant to seek treatment, or don't recognize the need for treatment, because their thought processes are impaired by the emotional problem. It is important to seek help as soon as the problems are detected.

How do we know if we are emotionally healthy? People who are emotionally healthy have problems, have down times, and sometimes have difficulty coping with their emotions. Yet they can understand and deal with reality. They can adapt to change and cope with stress. They have the capacity for love and concern and can work effectively to meet their basic needs. If we have these qualities, chances are that we are emotionally healthy.

LEARNING OBJECTIVES

Goal

You should be able to explain the goal of psychological health, the characteristics and behaviors of psychologically healthy people, coping mechanisms, and the symptoms and risk factors of mental illness and suicide.

Objectives

Upon completion of this lesson, you should be able to:

1. Explain the goal of psychological health, the characteristics and behaviors of psychologically healthy people, their coping mechanisms, sleep patterns, and communications with others.

2. Discuss the major psychological problem, risk factors and symptoms of suicide and its prevention.

KEY TERMS

Look for these items as you proceed through the lesson assignments. Be able to discuss them upon completion of this lesson.

emotional health
mental health
spiritual health
emotional intelligence
spiritual intelligence
culture
mood
optimism
altruism
autonomy
locus of control
assertive
rapid-eye-movement (REM) sleep
social isolation
social phobia
personality disorder
anxiety
mental disorder
depression
psychoneuroimmunology
anxiety disorders
phobia
panic attack
generalized anxiety disorder (GAD)
obsessive-compulsive disorder (OCD)
panic disorder
depressive disorders
major depression
bipolar disorder
seasonal affective disorder (SAD)
dysthymia
attention deficit/hyperactivity disorder (ADHD)
schizophrenia

TEXT FOCUS POINTS

The following focus points are designed to help you get the most from the text. Review them, then read the assignment. You may want to write notes to reinforce what you have learned.

Text: Hales, *An Invitation to Health*, Chapter 3, pp. 66–70, pp. 72–92, and pp. 98–102.

1. Explain the goal of psychological health. What are the characteristics of emotionally healthy people? Of mental (intellectual) health?

2. How can a psychologically healthy person find meaning in life, achieve a sense of control, and maintain a desired energy level?

3. List healthy and unhealthy coping mechanisms, and explain ways to create more positive and effective coping mechanisms in one's life.

4. Describe ways one can cope with loneliness and social anxieties, develop social skills, and get along with difficult people.

5. Discuss the major psychological problems experienced by members of our society.

6. Identify the symptoms and risk factors associated with depression, anxiety disorders, attention disorders, and schizophrenia.

7. What are the risk factors for suicide and what strategies help prevent suicide?

VIDEO FOCUS POINTS

The following focus points are designed to help you get the most from the video segment of this lesson. Review them, then watch the video. You may want to write notes to reinforce what you have learned.

Video: "Emotional Health"

1. What are some of the attributes of emotionally healthy people?

2. Describe some of the most common negative emotions and the way in which they can affect the individual.

3. Discuss some of the ways in which emotionally healthy people cope with negative emotions and conflict.

4. Explain the factors that put an individual at risk for suicide. Include the signs that would alert others to the fact that an individual may be thinking of suicide.

INDIVIDUAL HEALTH PLAN

This portion of the lesson is designed to enable you to use the information you have learned in your own life situation to improve the quality of your life. You should do any exercise assigned, complete the journal portion of the plan, then put this portion of the health plan into practice in your life.

> Complete the Self-Survey, "Is Something Wrong?" on page 79 of your textbook. Analyze your answers. If you feel that you could use some help, seek it at your college counseling center or other facility. Look at your coping mechanisms and general state of emotional well-being. If there are things that you wish to change, develop a plan for doing this. Use your journal to put your plan on paper where you can follow it and refer to it on a daily basis.

RELATED ACTIVITIES

These activities are not required unless your instructor assigns them. They are offered as suggestions to help you learn more about the material presented in this lesson.

> Interview some people that you consider emotionally healthy. Find out something about their lifestyles and how they cope with problems in life.

PRACTICE TEST

After reading the assignment and watching the video, you should be able to answer the Practice Test questions. Tests also include essay questions that are similar to the Text Focus Points and the Video Focus Points. When you have completed the Practice Test questions, turn to the Answer Key to score your answers.

Multiple-Choice

Select the one choice that best answers the question.

1. All of the following might express actions of a psychologically healthy person EXCEPT he or she __________.
   A. establishes ties with family
   B. holds others to higher levels of expectations than self
   C. pursues work or job that suits natural talents
   D. accepts own limitations as a reality of life

2. Which question would be the most meaningful to focus on in relation to positive emotional health in respect to life's emotions and feelings?
   A. The whys of your life
   B. The whos in your life
   C. The wheres in your life
   D. The hows of your life

3. A sustained emotional state that colors our view of the world for hours or days best describes __________.
   A. mood
   B. altruism
   C. autonomy
   D. self-esteem

4. One of the prime necessities in life related to the concept of love for mature adults is __________.
   A. we need to express love as well as receive love
   B. love is not necessarily a basic human need
   C. emotional health is less concerned with love than mental health
   D. all of the above are true regarding love

5. A major risk factor to disease and early death related to a lack of connectedness and social contact is known as __________.
   A. autonomy
   B. social isolation
   C. REM sleep
   D. shyness

6. The most common mental disorders in the United States are __________.
   A. anxiety disorders
   B. dependence disorders
   C. major depression
   D. dysthymia

7. All of the following might be warning signs of panic attack EXCEPT ________.
   A. racing heartbeat, breathing trouble, and chest pain
   B. fear of losing control of a given situation
   C. trembling or shaking
   D. a strong desire to commit suicide

8. All of the following are characteristic symptoms of phobias EXCEPT ________.
   A. excessive or irrational fear of object or situation
   B. intense anxiety and distress from exposure to object or situation
   C. lack of recognition of what the fear actually is about
   D. inability to function as usual in some social situations

9. All of the following are generally recognized treatments for anxiety disorders EXCEPT __________.
   A. psychotherapy
   B. behavioral therapy
   C. antianxiety drugs
   D. institutionalization

10. A compulsion is defined as which of the following?
    A. Exaggerated and persistent fear of something
    B. Repetitive behaviors performed according to certain routine
    C. Recurrent but senseless ideas, thoughts, impulses, or images
    D. Unexpected and unprovoked emotionally intense experiences

11. The most frequently prescribed drugs for bipolar disorder are __________.
    A. mood stabilizing drugs
    B. tranquilizers
    C. antidepressants
    D. stimulants

12. All of the following might be common characteristics of depression EXCEPT _________.
    A. childhood trauma increases vulnerability to depression
    B. occurs in 15–40% of college-age men and women
    C. renders one incapable of concentrating on work
    D. is similar to the "blues"

13. All of the following are types of depression EXCEPT __________.
    A. manic
    B. clinical
    C. schizophrenia
    D. major

14. Hyperactivity, impulsive behavior, and an easy distractibility in a child may all be signs of __________.
    A. depression
    B. suicidal tendencies
    C. attention deficit
    D. schizophrenia

15. Which of the following might be a typical behavior of a schizophrenic individual in the residual phase of his or her disease?
    A. Sees space aliens as a threat to the world
    B. Withdraws from friends and family
    C. Believes someone is sending them secret thoughts
    D. Acts strangely in social settings

16. Which of the following statements from a student might be the most significant warning sign for suicide?
    A. "I don't know what I'm doing and everything seems hopeless."
    B. "I don't know why but my parents just don't understand me."
    C. "I need a job and I can't seem to find one."
    D. "I'm angry and mad at the whole world."

17. Emotionally healthy people __________.
    A. frequently cope with depression
    B. usually see ways to overcome problems
    C. never experience failure
    D. always seem to be happy

18. That negative emotions affect individuals is evidenced by all the following symptoms EXCEPT __________.
    A. interruptions in sleep
    B. change in appetite
    C. feelings of intense despair
    D. ability to concentrate

19. Healthy ways of coping with negative emotions would be LEAST likely to include __________.
    A. maintaining self-esteem
    B. talking to others
    C. denying the emotions
    D. doing enjoyable activities

Fill-in-the-Blank

Insert the correct word or words in the blank for each item.

20. __________ __________ describes our ability to perceive reality as it is, to respond to its challenges, and to develop rational strategies for living.

21. A __________ is a more sustained emotional state that colors our view of the world for hours or days.

22. People who help others and give of themselves, thus promoting their own self-esteem, are said to be ___________.

23. People who communicate well with others and have a _______________ in their relationships tend to be healthier and happier.

24. __________ are inordinate fears of certain objects or situations.

25. ______________ is a mental illness whose origin is usually found in abnormalities of brain function or brain chemicals and may result in an impaired sense of reality.

26. Emotions that disrupt the balance of one's life are termed ________________.

27. Feelings of hopelessness, helplessness, and despair can increase the risk of ________________.

True-False

If the statement is true, write "T" to the left of the statement. If the statement (or any part of the statement) is false, write "F" to the left of the statement.

28. Short of seeking professional help, an individual can do little to cope with negative emotions.

29. Being able to talk about feelings of suicide with caring friends can temporarily lower an individual's probability of acting.

ANSWER KEY

The following provides the answers and references for the Practice Test questions. Focus Points are referenced using the following abbreviations:

T = Text and V = Video

	Answers	Learning Objectives	Focus Points	References
1.	B	1	T1	Hales, p. 68
2.	A	1	T1	Hales, p. 69
3.	A	1	T2	Hales, p. 72
4.	A	1	T3	Hales, p. 75
5.	B	2	T4	Hales, p. 76
6.	C	2	T5	Hales, p. 84
7.	D	2	T6	Hales, p. 83
8.	C	2	T6	Hales, p. 83
9.	D	2	T6	Hales, p. 84
10.	B	2	T6	Hales, p. 84
11.	A	2	T6	Hales, p. 87
12.	B	2	T6	Hales, p. 85
13.	C	2	T6	Hales, p. 84
14.	C	2	T6	Hales, p. 90
15.	D	2	T6	Hales, p. 92
16.	A	2	T7	Hales, p. 89
17.	B	1	V1	Video
18.	D	1	V2	Video
19.	C	1	V3	Video
20.	Mental health	1	T1	Hales, p. 68
21.	mood	1	T2	Hales, p. 72
22.	altruistic	1	T3	Hales, p. 75
23.	connectedness	1	T4	Hales, p. 76
24.	Phobias	2	T6	Hales, p. 83
25.	Schizophrenia	2	T6	Hales, p. 91
26.	negative	1	V2	Video
27.	suicide	2	V4	Video
28.	F	1	V2	Video
29.	T	2	V4	Video

Lesson 4

Intellectual Well-Being

Morale is self-esteem in action.

—Avery Weisman, M.D.

LESSON ASSIGNMENT

Review the following assignment in order to schedule your time appropriately. Pay careful attention; the titles and numbers of the textbook chapter, the telecourse guide lesson, and the video program may be different from one another.

Text:

Hales, *An Invitation to Health,*
Chapter 3, "Psychological Health," pp. 71–72 and pp. 92–102.

Video:

"Intellectual Well-Being"
from the series *Living with Health.*

OVERVIEW

Though many people equate intellect with education, the two are far from the same. Our intellect is the thinking, reasoning, problem-solving part of our consciousness. We all have it, no matter what our level of education. While our emotions allow us to feel, our intellect moderates these emotions and helps us to solve problems and to learn. Our emotions and our intellect work together to make us mentally healthy. If one or the other is not fully used, we lack quality of life and can even become mentally ill.

The ability to learn is critical to our health. We begin learning from birth and continue to learn throughout life. We model the behavior of others. We learn through trial and error, and we remember past experiences. Our behavior and health practices result from what we have learned from our life experiences.

In order to maintain good health, it is imperative that we use our intellect to solve problems and make good decisions about our health. To make these decisions, we must be sure we clearly understand the problems. Too often, we try to solve problems before we really understand them. Look at life's problems from several directions before you try to solve them. Once we understand the problems, we develop strategies for solving them. An important point here is the knowledge that there is rarely only one solution. We must open our minds to the idea that there are various strategies available to us. We may try one that doesn't work. Don't give up—try another one.

The final stage of problem solving is decision making, a critical part of the process! All of us have known people who couldn't seem to make a decision. They could understand the problem, develop strategies, but just didn't take that final step. People like this are frequently unhappy because others step in and make their decisions for them. Don't be one of these people. Make your own decisions regarding your health. Then—be sure and take action on your decision!

A most important part of our being is our self-concept, or the perception we have about ourselves. Our self-concept evolves throughout our lives, based on our evaluation of ourselves and what other people think. Both our emotions and our intellect play an intertwining role in development of a positive self-concept. Self-concept is crucial to our mental health. If we do not have a realistic, positive self-concept, we are not healthy, no matter how healthy we are physically. In order to have high self-esteem, or a good sense of worth and dignity, we must have a positive self-concept. This positive self-concept, with its resulting high self-esteem, shapes our self-efficacy, the confidence that we have in ourselves to accomplish things in our lives and take care of our health.

We have spent time discussing the positive aspects of intellect and emotions, but sometimes, during our lives and those of ones we care about, things don't come together in a positive fashion. For whatever reason, there are problems we can't solve or feelings that we can't cope with. In the past, and sometimes even now, people are hesitant to seek help for mental problems. Somehow, seeking mental help may have a stigma that seeking physical help does not have. This is very unfortunate, because it is crucial for people to seek professional help when they have mental or emotional problems. Good counseling or therapy can aid an individual in returning to a fully functioning, high quality of life. If you or someone you know is experiencing depression, problems with relationships, eating or sleeping problems, mood swings, or other signs of emotional problems, make a decision at once to get help. With help, we can overcome these problems and lead a healthy, happy life.

Together, our intellect and emotions are the most powerful tools we have for building and maintaining our healthy lifestyles. It is imperative that we use them well.

LEARNING OBJECTIVES

Goal

You should be able to explain the relationship of needs, values, and goals to psychological health, self-esteem, the brain, and different therapeutic approaches to treatment.

Objectives

Upon completion of this lesson, you should be able to:

1. Discuss the relationship of needs, feelings, values, goals, and self-esteem.
2. Explain the brain as the "master control center of the body," and describe the various therapeutic treatments.
3. Explain the roles that learning, problem solving, decision making, dealing with failure, self-concept, and self-esteem play in health and wellness.

KEY TERMS

Look for these items as you proceed through the lesson assignments. Be able to discuss them upon completion of this lesson.

self-actualization
values
moral
self-esteem
neuropsychiatry
glia
neurons
axon
axon terminal
dendrite
neurotransmitter
nucleus
receptors
synapse
reuptake
certified social worker
licensed clinical social worker (LCSW)
psychiatric nurse
psychiatrist
psychologist
marriage and family therapy
psychodynamics
psychotherapy
behavior therapy
cognitive therapy
interpersonal therapy (IPT)
psychiatric drug therapy

TEXT FOCUS POINTS

The following focus points are designed to help you get the most from the text. Review them, then read the assignment. You may want to write notes to reinforce what you have learned.

Text: Hales, *An Invitation to Health*, Chapter 3, pp. 71–72 and pp. 92–102.

1. Discuss the relationship of needs, feelings, values, and goals to psychological health.

2. Define self-esteem and list some strategies for increasing one's self-esteem.

3. Explain why neuropsychiatrists consider the brain to be the "master control center of the body" and the last frontier in their research.

4. Identify and briefly describe a variety of modern approaches used by professional therapists.

VIDEO FOCUS POINTS

The following focus points are designed to help you get the most from the video segment of this lesson. Review them, then watch the video. You may want to write notes to reinforce what you have learned.

Video: "Intellectual Well-Being"

1. What roles do learning, problem solving, and decision making play in health and well-being?

2. Discuss self-concept and self-esteem.

3. Why is it important to be able to deal with failure in a positive manner?

INDIVIDUAL HEALTH PLAN

This portion of the lesson is designed to enable you to use the information you have learned in your own life situation to improve the quality of your life. You should do any exercise assigned, complete the journal portion of the plan, then put this portion of the health plan into practice in your life.

> Think back on some major problem or issue you have had to address. List the steps you took to come to the conclusion. Were these successful? If not, what could you do differently next time?

RELATED ACTIVITIES

These activities are not required unless your instructor assigns them. They are offered as suggestions to help you learn more about the material presented in this lesson.

> Visit a community mental health resource, such as a crisis intervention center. Become familiar with the role such resources play in a community.

PRACTICE TEST

After reading the assignment and watching the video, you should be able to answer the Practice Test questions. Tests also include essay questions that are similar to the Text Focus Points and the Video Focus Points. When you have completed the Practice Test questions, turn to the Answer Key to score your answers.

Multiple-Choice

Select the one choice that best answers the question.

1. Which of the following situations would represent a terminal value?
   A. Loyalty to country
   B. Earning a college degree
   C. Serving God
   D. Being a good parent

2. All of the following might be common characteristics of an individual with low self-esteem EXCEPT a __________.
   A. person who was abused as a child
   B. person who lived in a rural environment
   C. person who is an alcoholic
   D. person who is chronically anxious

3. Which of the following therapists is licensed to prescribe drug medications?
   A. Psychologists
   B. Psychiatrists
   C. Licensed clinical social workers
   D. All of the above can prescribe medications

4. The final, important step in the problem-solving process is to __________.
   A. select strategies
   B. make a decision
   C. verify the decision
   D. define the problem

5. Self-concept includes individuals' perceptions of their __________.
   A. lovableness
   B. partners' abilities
   C. self-esteem
   D. strengths and weaknesses

6. Failure must be viewed as a __________.
   A. step in the learning process
   B. very personal thing
   C. reflection of oneself
   D. sign of not trying hard enough

Fill-in-the-Blank

Insert the correct word or words in the blank for each item.

7. _______ are the criteria by which we evaluate things, peoples, events, and ourselves.

8. _________ therapy involves identification of an individual's beliefs and attitudes and the modification of negative thought patterns toward more positive thought patterns.

9. The intellect is the force that causes people to be able to solve problems and make decisions in the process of ________________.

10. Being able to accept credit for a job well done is an example of high ________________.

True-False

If the statement is true, write "T" to the left of the statement. If the statement (or any part of the statement) is false, write "F" to the left of the statement.

11. Using one's intuition is the final, important step in problem solving.

12. Self-esteem describes a person's feelings of worth and dignity.

13. People who are expanding their experiences will probably experience some failures.

ANSWER KEY

The following provides the answers and references for the Practice Test questions. Focus Points are referenced using the following abbreviations:

T = Text and V = Video

	Answers	Learning Objectives	Focus Points	References
1.	B	1	T1	Hales, p. 71
2.	B	1	T2	Hales, p. 71
3.	B	2	T4	Hales, p. 93
4.	C	3	V1	Video
5.	D	3	V2	Video
6.	A	3	V3	Video
7.	Values	1	T1	Hales, p. 71
8.	Cognitive	2	T4	Hales, p. 94
9.	learning	3	V1	Video
10.	self-esteem	3	V2	Video
11.	F	3	V1	Video
12.	T	3	V2	Video
13.	T	3	V3	Video

Lesson 5

Fitness and Exercise

You will begin to touch heaven, Jonathan, in the moment that you touch perfect speed. And that isn't flying a thousand miles an hour, or a million, or flying at the speed of light. Because any number is a limit, and perfection doesn't have limits. Perfect speed, my son, is being there.

—Richard Bach, *Jonathan Livingston Seagull*

LESSON ASSIGNMENT

Review the following assignment in order to schedule your time appropriately. Pay careful attention; the titles and numbers of the textbook chapter, the telecourse guide lesson, and the video program may be different from one another.

Text:

Hales, *An Invitation to Health,*
Chapter 4, "The Joy of Fitness," pp. 103–142.

Video:

"Fitness and Exercise"
from the series *Living with Health.*

OVERVIEW

As the old seagull tells Jonathon, the important thing is being there. So it is with fitness and exercise—the important thing is that you are doing something physical on a regular basis. It is not important for you to become a marathon runner or run the four-minute mile. It is important for you to get enough exercise to keep your cardiovascular system in good shape and to give you the strength and endurance to do the things you want. It is no secret that people who are physically fit are healthier, more productive, and have a higher quality of life than those who are not. We also know that almost anyone can engage is some kind of exercise program. The mystery is why only about 20 percent of Americans engage in even moderate intensity exercise.

Some of the answers may lie in our American way of life. We have all kinds of technology to make our life easier. Most of us have sedentary jobs that we drive to and from, and too many of us come home from our sedentary jobs to spend the evening on the couch in front of the television. For recreation, we go to movies or to a spectator sporting event, where the only exercise we get is walking to the concession stand for popcorn. Consider also, this is the model that our children are seeing. Is it any wonder that our "couch potato" image is being passed on to the next generation? We are part of the generation that can change all this, and make ourselves a generation of healthy people, for future generations to model. Besides, fitness is fun! It feels good to have the energy to do the things we want to. It is fun to feel in control of this part of our life.

If you are willing to invest even three hours a week in a fitness program, you will see significant results. A program of vigorous walking for thirty minutes, three to five times a week, alternating with simple strength building exercises, will accomplish that level of fitness required for good health. If you don't want to or can't walk for exercise, then bicycle riding, swimming, or other aerobic activity will accomplish the same thing. A regular program like this will give you other benefits as well. Exercise helps us cope with stress, makes us feel more healthy emotionally, gives us a feeling of self-esteem and self-efficacy, can be a social activity, and gives our spiritual self a lift as well. This investment of ourselves helps us achieve all the dimensions of health.

Now that we are all convinced and ready to start our exercise program, let's discuss the healthy way to start. First, start slowly! If you have been inactive for several years, are more than thirty years old, or suffer from a chronic health problem, examination by a physician is very important. Your physician can order tests that will help ensure that you are ready for an exercise program. If, after this lesson, you are still unsure how to begin your own program, consult your instructor, a staff member of your college health center, or some other health or physical education professional. The only financial investment that you have to make is in a good pair of suitable shoes designed for the activity you will choose. Remember that just as improvement will begin very soon, conditioning is lost very soon if you stop your program. Make a pledge to yourself to keep your program going. You owe it to yourself!

So get a checkup, put on those shoes, and hit the road! If you think you might need a little extra motivation and help, enroll in a class at a college near you or join a good fitness club.

LEARNING OBJECTIVES

Goal

You should be able to describe the benefits of exercise, the components of fitness, and explain the components and modifications of an exercise program.

Objectives

Upon completion of this lesson, you should be able to:

1. Describe the physical and psychological benefits of regular exercise and the components of physical fitness.

2. Discuss the components of a plan for a regular exercise program, the principles of nutrition, safety, products to be considered, and the risks of anabolic steroid use.

KEY TERMS

Look for these items as you proceed through the lesson assignments. Be able to discuss them upon completion of this lesson.

physical fitness
flexibility
cardiovascular fitness
aerobic exercise
anaerobic exercise
strength
endurance
conditioning
osteoporosis
endorphins
resting heart rate
target heart rate
overloading
isometric
isotonic
isokinetic
sets
rep or repetition
ergogenic aid
cross-training
aerobic circuit training
acute injuries
overuse injuries
overtrain

TEXT FOCUS POINTS

The following focus points are designed to help you get the most from the text. Review them, then read the assignment. You may want to write notes to reinforce what you have learned.

Text: Hales, *An Invitation to Health,* Chapter 4, pp. 103–142.

1. List the components of physical fitness and explain each.

2. What are the benefits of exercise as a part of one's health promotion program? How does exercise prevent disease?

3. Describe actions and exercises that can improve flexibility, cardiovascular fitness, and muscular strength and endurance.

4. Discuss the risks and dangers of anabolic steroid use.

5. Develop a total fitness program. Include principles of nutrition, safety, and appropriate fitness products and programs.

VIDEO FOCUS POINTS

The following focus points are designed to help you get the most from the video segment of this lesson. Review them, then watch the video. You may want to write notes to reinforce what you have learned.

Video: "Fitness and Exercise"

1. What are some of the physical benefits of exercise? Include the components of fitness or, as it is also known, "fitness for health."

2. What factors need to be considered when designing and beginning an exercise program?

3. In what ways is progression important in an exercise program?

4. Describe some of the mental and emotional benefits of exercising.

INDIVIDUAL HEALTH PLAN

This portion of the lesson is designed to enable you to use the information you have learned in your own life situation to improve the quality of your life. You should do any exercise assigned, complete the journal portion of the plan, then put this portion of the health plan into practice in your life.

> Complete the Self-Survey, "What's Your Physical Activity I.Q." on page 114 of your text. Then, in the journal you are keeping, track your physical activity and your physical exercise for a week or more. From this information, and using what you have learned in this lesson, develop a program of regular exercise for yourself. Write the plan in your journal, so that you are able to modify it as you need to. Once you have developed a plan that suits your needs and abilities, begin or continue your regular exercise program.

RELATED ACTIVITIES

These activities are not required unless your instructor assigns them. They are offered as suggestions to help you learn more about the material presented in this lesson.

1. Visit several health clubs and fitness facilities and compare and evaluate their programs.

2. Interview several people of varying ages and levels of fitness. Ask them about their fitness programs. What did you think about the components of their program and the quality of it?

PRACTICE TEST

After reading the assignment and watching the video, you should be able to answer the Practice Test questions. Tests also include essay questions that are similar to the Text Focus Points and the Video Focus Points. When you have completed the Practice Test questions, turn to the Answer Key to score your answers.

Multiple-Choice

Select the one choice that best answers the question.

1. The ability to move the muscles and joints through their natural range of motion is an example of __________.
   A. flexibility
   B. stamina
   C. strength
   D. endurance

2. All of the following are potential benefits of a regular exercise program EXCEPT __________.
   A. strengthening and thickening of heart muscles
   B. having denser bone structure
   C. maintaining weight more efficiently
   D. having a higher clotting capability in the bloodstream

3. Isotonic muscular strength training is best achieved by working with __________.
   A. high resistance with many repetitions
   B. high resistance with few repetitions
   C. low resistance with many repetitions
   D. low resistance with few repetitions

4. Anabolic steroid use has been associated with __________.
   A. heart abnormalities
   B. high blood pressure
   C. psychological abnormalities
   D. all of the above

5. After exercise, the best choice of action to prevent dehydration is __________.
   A. drinking water
   B. drinking a sports drink to return lost minerals
   C. drinking a juice drink to return used sugar
   D. taking salt tablets

6. While playing a game of basketball, you come down on the foot of another player and severely twist your ankle. This is an example of __________.
   A. an overuse injury
   B. an acute injury
   C. overtraining
   D. cross-training injury

7. The components of fitness include all the following EXCEPT __________.
   A. strength
   B. skill
   C. endurance
   D. flexibility

8. In designing a fitness program, one of the most important considerations is the individual's __________.
   A. initial fitness level
   B. height
   C. skill level
   D. schedule

9. Progression in an exercise program is important to __________.
   A. maintain health benefits
   B. improve fitness levels
   C. increase skill levels
   D. feel good

10. Mental benefits of exercise include all the following EXCEPT __________.
   A. sense of well-being
   B. cardiovascular health
   C. mental alertness
   D. positive attitude

Fill-in-the-Blank

Insert the correct word or words in the blank for each item.

11. The length of time muscular work can be maintained is a measure of muscular _____________.

12. Training the muscles by moving greater amounts than the muscles ordinarily move is known as the _______________ principle.

13. Sprains, bruises, pulled muscles, or injuries as a result of sudden trauma are known as _________ injuries.

14. It is important to design an exercise program that builds endurance, flexibility, and ______________.

True-False

If the statement is true, write "T" to the left of the statement. If the statement (or any part of the statement) is false, write "F" to the left of the statement.

15. Progression in an exercise program is just one of the ways to increase fitness level.

ANSWER KEY

The following provides the answers and references for the Practice Test questions. Focus Points are referenced using the following abbreviations:

T = Text and V = Video

	Answers	Learning Objectives	Focus Points	References
1.	A	1	T1	Hales, p. 107
2.	D	1	T2	Hales, p. 110
3.	B	1	T3	Hales, p. 125
4.	D	2	T4	Hales, p. 127
5.	A	2	T5	Hales, p. 136
6.	B	2	T5	Hales, p. 133
7.	B	1	V1	Video
8.	A	2	V2	Video
9.	B	2	V3	Video
10.	B	1	V4	Video
11.	endurance	1	T1	Hales, p. 106
12.	overloading	1	T3	Hales, p. 125
13.	acute	2	T5	Hales, p. 135
14.	strength	2	V2	Video
15.	F..	2	V3	Video

Lesson 6

Diet and Nutrition

We're not sure whether vegetables are macho enough.

—Arlyn Hackett

LESSON ASSIGNMENT

Review the following assignment in order to schedule your time appropriately. Pay careful attention; the titles and numbers of the textbook chapter, the telecourse guide lesson, and the video program may be different from one another.

Text:

Hales, *An Invitation to Health*,
Chapter 5, "Personal Nutrition," pp. 144–186.

Video:

"Diet and Nutrition"
from the series *Living with Health*.

OVERVIEW

We probably think more about diet and nutrition today than ever before in our history. However, do we really practice better nutrition principles now that we know what we should be eating? If we look at the crowds in local farmers' markets buying fresh fruit and vegetables, we would say yes. However if we check out the lines in the neighborhood fast food establishments, the answer would be absolutely not. Then, if we followed you around the grocery store, the answer would be ????

Thanks to advanced technology, higher standards of living, and an abundance of nutrition information, Americans have access to very good nutrition. Yet, for a variety of reasons, many of us are malnourished. We certainly eat plenty; frequently too much. Unfortunately, too often we make poor choices in our selection of food. We tend to eat foods that are high in saturated fat, salt, and refined sugar, rather than choosing fruits, vegetables, and foods high in fiber and low in fats. Even worse, children eat just like adults, thus increasing their risk of nutrition-related illness.

Many people complain that good nutrition is expensive or too much trouble. Actually, a healthy diet can be far less expensive than a poor one and just as easy to prepare. Fast food and "junk" food are certainly not cheap. Few of the rich, refined foods are easy to prepare. Good nutrition involves an understanding of foods that are healthy and some simple planning of daily intake. Plainly stated, we need to increase our consumption of complex carbohydrates, decrease our consumption of protein, and limit our fats, salt, and refined sugar. Translated into foods, this means more fruits, vegetables, whole grain and enriched breads and pasta, and less meats, fast foods, salt, fats, and high calorie desserts. It also means steaming, baking, or broiling foods instead of frying them or covering them with gravy or rich sauces.

Even those who eat out can improve their nutritional status by using good judgment in food selection. Most restaurants (even our favorite fast food establishments) are beginning to offer more health conscious options on their menus. The more we choose and request these healthy foods, the more will be offered. All of us can eat a more healthy diet and enjoy it. We can get these foods in most supermarkets and restaurants. We do not need to go to extremes of shopping at a health food store to ensure good nutrition.

We have all the elements of a healthy diet that ensures good nutrition easily available to us if we simply make good choices. You know what to eat—the choice is now yours!

LEARNING OBJECTIVES

Goal

You should be able to discuss nutrition and the principles, strategies, and food choices involved in achieving a healthy diet.

Objectives

Upon completion of this lesson, you should be able to:

1. Explain the term "nutrition," discuss the nutrients necessary for a healthy body, and explain the USDA Food Guide Pyramid as a guide to good nutrition.

2. Describe the role of good nutrition and food safety in preventing disease and promoting health.

3. Discuss various approaches used to achieve a balanced healthy diet, and basic principles, strategies, and skills important in achieving good nutrition.

KEY TERMS

Look for these items as you proceed through the lesson assignments. Be able to discuss them upon completion of this lesson.

nutrition
nutrients
protein
carbohydrates
simple carbohydrates
complex carbohydrates
fiber
saturated fat
unsaturated fat
trans fats
cholesterol
vitamins
fat-soluble vitamins
water-soluble vitamins
minerals
antioxidants
hemoglobin
phytochemicals
crucifers
indoles
calorie
lacto-vegetarians
ovo-lacto-vegetarians
vegans
complementary proteins
complete proteins
amino acids
incomplete proteins
food toxicologists
organic
irradiation
additives
E. coli
listeria
botulism
food allergies

TEXT FOCUS POINTS

The following focus points are designed to help you get the most from the text. Review them, then read the assignment. You may want to write notes to reinforce what you have learned.

Text: Hales, *An Invitation to Health*, Chapter 5, pp. 144–186.

1. Explain what is meant by the term "nutrition." List and define the basic nutrients necessary for a healthy body, and give examples of foods containing these nutrients.

2. List the United States Department of Agriculture (USDA) recommendations for healthy eating. How does one use the new food labels to help achieve these recommendations?

3. Describe the USDA Food Guide Pyramid and explain its significance for nutrition and recommended servings of each type of food. Include the importance of water in the diet and the amount needed daily. How do the requirements for young children and older adults differ from those of the younger adult?

4. Compare the different forms of fat, and list the ones preferable for use when attempting to keep one's cholesterol levels low.

5. Explain the contributions of good nutrition to the prevention of heart disease and cancer.

6. Discuss the use of vitamin and mineral supplements, including what types of people need which supplements, as well as the potential dangers involved in megadoses.

7. Analyze the various alternative and ethnic diets and describe the advantages and disadvantages of each. Include "fast food" in your discussion.

8. What are the advantages and risks of pesticides? of additives?

9. Describe the source, symptoms, and preventions of the most common foodborne infections. Include the contribution of food safety to personal health.

VIDEO FOCUS POINTS

The following focus points are designed to help you get the most from the video segment of this lesson. Review them, then watch the video. You may want to write notes to reinforce what you have learned.

Video: "Diet and Nutrition"

1. What are important "tips" or principles for menu planning and selecting food wisely in the supermarket?

2. What is meant by the idea of "reordering the American diet"?

3. Discuss ways in which food can be prepared to lower the intake of fats, salt, and refined sugar and to increase its nutrition.

INDIVIDUAL HEALTH PLAN

This portion of the lesson is designed to enable you to use the information you have learned in your own life situation to improve the quality of your life. You should do any exercise assigned, complete the journal portion of the plan, then put this portion of the health plan into practice in your life.

> Using the Self-Survey, "Rate Your Diet," on pages 161–162 of your textbook, keep a journal of your dietary intake for a week. Evaluate it. Is this your normal diet? How do you rank yourself on your intake of healthy foods? Does your diet contain too much cholesterol and saturated fats, salt, sugar, and "empty" calories? Using this evaluation, plan a food strategy that will provide you with good nutrition, and that you will be willing to follow for an extended time. As you do this, use the USDA Food Guide Pyramid as your guide.
>
> Once you have written your plan, try it out for two weeks. Reevaluate it and consider making this a permanent part of your lifestyle.

RELATED ACTIVITIES

These activities are not required unless your instructor assigns them. They are offered as suggestions to help you learn more about the material presented in this lesson.

1. Go to a grocery store and observe what people are buying. Compare and evaluate the quality of their diets, based on their food selections.

2. Go to a cafeteria or buffet and observe how people are eating. Note whether the children are eating like their parents. Evaluate their diets as though they eat all the time as you are seeing them eat now.

PRACTICE TEST

After reading the assignment and watching the video, you should be able to answer the Practice Test questions. Tests also include essay questions that are similar to the Text Focus Points and the Video Focus Points. When you have completed the Practice Test questions, turn to the Answer Key to score your answers.

Multiple-Choice

Select the one choice that best answers the question.

1. All of the following are functions of fiber in our diet EXCEPT __________.
   A. lowers blood cholesterol
   B. does not decrease risk of colon cancer
   C. increases bulk in large intestine waste elimination
   D. supplies calories for energy

2. Fats derived primarily from animal sources are referred to as __________.
   A. polyunsaturated
   B. monounsaturated
   C. saturated
   D. hydrogenated

3. Organic compounds that the body needs in small amounts to perform regulatory functions are known as __________.
   A. protein
   B. carbohydrates
   C. vitamins
   D. minerals

4. Antioxidants help to defend the body against the development of disease-causing compounds known as __________.
   A. atherosclerosis
   B. free radicals
   C. sodium
   D. cholesterol

5. Foods to be limited at the top of the food pyramid are __________.
   A. breads, cereals, and grains
   B. meat and meat substitutes
   C. fats, oils, and sweets
   D. all of the above should be equally limited

6. The label standard for determining the amount of any nutrient needed on a daily basis is __________.
   A. recommended dietary allowances
   B. recommended daily allowances
   C. daily value
   D. food guides

7. A good example of complementary proteins combined to form complete proteins from individual incomplete proteins might be __________.
   A. beans and rice
   B. carrots and sweet peas
   C. eggs and ham
   D. watermelon and bananas

8. Foods termed as organic supposedly have not been exposed to __________.
   A. additives
   B. irradiation
   C. hormones or antibiotics
   D. commercial chemicals

9. The following could be sources of foodborne bacterial infections EXCEPT ____.
   A. milk left out of the refrigerator for two hours
   B. barbecued chicken that has been placed back in a pre-cooked marinade sauce
   C. raw eggs used in salad dressing
   D. wooden cutting boards washed in hot soapy water

10. Healthy nutrition and food selection __________.
   A. becomes quite expensive
   B. involves careful choices
   C. seems difficult to achieve
   D. tends to be boring

11. Americans typically eat meals that contain too few __________.
   A. meat products
   B. breads
   C. milk products
   D. vegetables

Fill-in-the-Blank

Insert the correct word or words in the blank for each item.

12. ________________ fats are those found in vegetable oils, such as corn, soybean, safflower, and sesame.

13. Naturally occurring inorganic compounds that are needed in small amounts to perform essential functions are known as ___________.

14. When evaluating meat and dairy products, of particular concern are the calories that come from ______.

15. One of the healthiest ways to prepare vegetables is ________________.

True-False

If the statement is true, write "T" to the left of the statement. If the statement (or any part of the statement) is false, write "F" to the left of the statement.

16. Eating foods that are high in nutrition is expensive.

17. It is important to begin to consider vegetables and grains, instead of meat, as the primary focus of the plate.

18. Herbs and spices contain so much sodium that they are not a good substitute for salt.

ANSWER KEY

The following provides the answers and references for the Practice Test questions. Focus Points are referenced using the following abbreviations:
T = Text and V = Video

	Answers	Learning Objectives	Focus Points	References
1.	D	2	T5	Hales, p. 148
2.	C	2	T4	Hales, p. 150
3.	C	1	T1	Hales, p. 152
4.	B	3	T6	Hales, p. 157
5.	C	1	T3	Hales, p. 160
6.	D	1	T2	Hales, p. 160
7.	A	3	T7	Hales, p. 176
8.	D	3	T8	Hales, p. 179
9.	D	2	T9	Hales, p. 182
10.	B	3	V1	Video
11.	D	3	V2	Video
12.	Polyunsaturated	2	T4	Hales, p. 150
13.	minerals	1	T1	Hales, p. 152
14.	fat	3	V1	Video
15.	steaming	3	V3	Video
16.	F	3	V1	Video
17.	T	3	V2	Video
18.	F	3	V3	Video

Lesson 7

Weight Management

Some weight-loss plans are based on poor science or no science, and many on witchcraft.

—Peter D. Wood, D.Sc. Ph.D.

LESSON ASSIGNMENT

Review the following assignment in order to schedule your time appropriately. Pay careful attention; the titles and numbers of the textbook chapter, the telecourse guide lesson, and the video program may be different from one another.

Text:

Hales, *An Invitation to Health,*
Chapter 6, "Eating Patterns and Problems," pp. 188–215.

Video:

"Weight Management"
from the series *Living with Health.*

OVERVIEW

Have you noticed how many new diet books are being written, and how every magazine on the newsstand has a diet article every month? Does that tell you something? Americans are obsessed with dieting and everything that goes with it. Many people try every fad diet that comes out, only to lose the same twenty or thirty pounds over and over in a yo-yo pattern that gets them nowhere. Most of the fad diets are useless in the long run, and many are actually dangerous.

The obsession with thinness has even given us two relatively new disease conditions related to diet and self-concept: anorexia nervosa and bulimia. Both are fairly new to medicine and are a result of an obsession with thinness. These are very serious problems which have resulted in many deaths, particularly in young women.

There are many reasons for overweight, and we know that obesity raises our risks for many health problems. Most of us who are overweight know this and are concerned with how to lose the excess weight and keep it off. The "bottom line" is that we must expend more calories than we take in, and do so in a healthy way. We must also change our eating patterns and our lifestyles over the long term, not simply think in terms of weeks or months. We must also believe that we can do it. This is a matter of self-efficacy and self-esteem.

The key to losing weight and keeping it off is very familiar to all of us—a well-balanced diet, low in fats and simple sugars, combined with a good exercise program. If that sounds familiar, it should. The same fruits, vegetables, fiber, and complex carbohydrates that are essential to good nutrition are the drivers for a healthy weight-loss diet. We should be eating the healthy foods recommended for good nutrition and be leaving off the high calorie, high fat, and empty calorie foods that increase our weight and cholesterol levels. Along with this, a sound exercise program is essential. Remember what we learned about expending more calories than we take in! There is no doubt that explaining the principles of weight management is much more simple than actually doing it. But once you get started, it gets easier. It also helps to take it one day at a time, but know you are making lifestyle changes for the long term.

It is very important not to be misled by fad diets that promise quick weight loss or magic results. These only get you into trouble. What you are trying to accomplish is a relatively steady weight loss of one to two pounds a week, and an increase in your fitness level through your exercise program.

A very important thing to remember in all this is that your value as a person is not related to how much you weigh! Yes, you will be happier and healthier if you attain your goals in body composition and fitness level, but do not let this be the thing that you base your whole self-concept on. If you truly believe your value as a person is unrelated to your body composition, you will actually have an easier time with weight loss.

For those who are underweight, the same basic principles apply. In order to gain weight in a healthy way, you should increase your intake of the higher calorie foods in a diet based on good nutrition. You should still avoid the high protein or high fat diets, which can be dangerous. Exercise is a key to this program as well.

The principles you are learning apply whether you are overweight, underweight, or just right. A nutritious, well-balanced diet combined with a good exercise program is important for everyone.

LEARNING OBJECTIVES

Goal

You should be able to discuss weight management, problems of weight management, and successful weight management.

Objectives

Upon completion of this lesson, you should be able to:

1. Describe factors involved in obesity, means by which ideal body weight is determined, and health problems related to weight management problems and eating disorders.

2. Compare healthy and unhealthy approaches to weight control and the risks that may be related to dieting.

KEY TERMS

Look for these items as you proceed through the lesson assignments. Be able to discuss them upon completion of this lesson.

body-mass index
skin calipers
hydrostatic weighing
basal metabolic rate (BMR)
calorie
hunger
appetite
satiety
set-point theory
binge eating
eating disorders
anorexia nervosa
bulimia nervosa/bulimia
obesity

TEXT FOCUS POINTS

The following focus points are designed to help you get the most from the text. Review them, then read the assignment. You may want to write notes to reinforce what you have learned.

Text: Hales, *An Invitation to Health*, Chapter 6, pp. 188–215.

1. Describe three different methods for determining an individual's ideal body weight.

2. Explain several factors that influence food consumption and body composition.

3. Identify and describe the symptoms and dangers associated with abnormal eating behaviors and eating disorders.

4. What is obesity? What roles do genetics, lifestyle, and overeating play in determining whether an individual becomes obese?

5. Discuss approaches to weight loss for individuals who are mildly, moderately, and severely obese. Describe some practical, healthy ways to lose weight.

6. Explain how health problems can be caused by fad diets.

VIDEO FOCUS POINTS

The following focus points are designed to help you get the most from the video segment of this lesson. Review them, then watch the video. You may want to write notes to reinforce what you have learned.

Video: "Weight Management"

1. Explain the various aspects of the risks of overweight. What are some of the causes of overweight?

2. Describe some considerations in planning a weight-loss diet.

3. Why is exercise important in weight management? What kind of exercise program should be designed?

4. Discuss the causes and dangers of anorexia nervosa and bulimia.

INDIVIDUAL HEALTH PLAN

This portion of the lesson is designed to enable you to use the information you have learned in your own life situation to improve the quality of your life. You should do any exercise assigned, complete the journal portion of the plan, then put this portion of the health plan into practice in your life.

> Complete the Self-Survey, "Do You Know How to Lose Weight?" on pages 207–208. Calculate your body mass index and your ideal weight. Using these, your diet for a week from your journal, and your exercise plan, assess your need to change your body weight, your food intake, or your exercise plan. In your journal, discuss your findings and write out a plan for improving or maintaining your diet/exercise program. Try out the program you have planned for a few weeks and evaluate your progress.

RELATED ACTIVITIES

These activities are not required unless your instructor assigns them. They are offered as suggestions to help you learn more about the material presented in this lesson.

1. Compare the nutritional value of several different fad diets to one based on good nutrition. Evaluate your findings.

2. Visit several weight-loss centers and find out about their programs. Compare them and evaluate your findings.

3. Talk to someone who is recovering from or fighting anorexia nervosa or bulimia. Ask them about their perceptions of their problem, their self-concept, their goal for weight, etc.

PRACTICE TEST

After reading the assignment and watching the video, you should be able to answer the Practice Test questions. Tests also include essay questions that are similar to the Text Focus Points and the Video Focus Points. When you have completed the Practice Test questions, turn to the Answer Key to score your answers.

Multiple-Choice

Select the one choice that best answers the question.

1. The method of body fat determination known as hydrostatic weighing works off the principle that __________.
   A. a pound of muscle weighs more than a pound of fat
   B. fat is stored in various body regions
   C. lean muscle has more isotopes present
   D. muscle tissue is denser than fat tissue

2. The definition of hunger is __________.
   A. the fear of not having food
   B. the physiological drive to consume food
   C. the need for food determined by stomach contractions
   D. the psychological desire for food

3. All of the following are common practices associated with compulsive overeating EXCEPT __________.
   A. a history of failed diets
   B. using food for depression or loneliness
   C. eating food very slowly at meals
   D. eating without regard to hunger or taste

4. All of the following are potential warning signs of anorexia nervosa EXCEPT __________.
   A. an intense fear of gaining weight
   B. a distorted view of body image
   C. breakthrough bleeding between menstrual cycles
   D. refusal to maintain normal body weight

5. Obese men have a higher risk of developing all of the following diseases EXCEPT __________.
   A. heart disease
   B. hypertension
   C. cirrhosis
   D. colon cancer

6. All of the following are reasons dieting alone as a method of weight loss tends to fail most the time EXCEPT __________.
   A. diets only consider the calories consumed, which is only half the problem
   B. diets have an endpoint, so people return to eating patterns that support weight gain
   C. diets take so long that people don't usually lose the amount of weight that they desire
   D. diets rarely allow for setbacks, thus setting the individual up for failure from the start

7. All of the following are potential signs of dangerous or fraudulent weight-loss programs EXCEPT __________.
   A. they claim that their diets will eliminate cellulite
   B. they promote weight loss based on pills that block starches
   C. they assert that there are no health risks involved
   D. they guarantee a weight loss of one pound a week

8. Reasons for overweight include all the following EXCEPT __________.
   A. availability of fatty food
   B. increased health knowledge
   C. sedentary lifestyle
   D. modern technology

9. In planning a diet to lose weight, it is important to consider all the following EXCEPT __________.
   A. reducing the fastest way
   B. losing weight gradually
   C. increasing exercise
   D. maintaining weight loss

10. Exercise is important to a weight-loss program because of all the following EXCEPT __________.
    A. metabolism is increased
    B. energy level is improved
    C. lethargy is increased
    D. body shape is improved

11. An important causal factor associated with anorexia nervosa and bulimia nervosa is __________.
    A. being overweight
    B. having a low self-esteem
    C. lacking appetite
    D. being underweight

Fill-in-the-Blank

Insert the correct word or words in the blank for each item.

12. The number of calories your body needs at rest to maintain body function is known as _______ ____________ _______.

13. The eating disorder that usually involves repeated bingeing and purging of food is known as ___________ ___________.

14. Many diet hucksters claim that their diets can eliminate __________, a term used to describe certain fatty tissue.

15. Two major causes of obesity are diets high in fat and lifestyles that are _______________.

16. A weight management program must include not only dietary modifications but also _________________.

True-False

If the statement is true, write "T" to the left of the statement. If the statement (or any part of the statement) is false, write "F" to the left of the statement.

17. A successful weight-loss program involves long-term dietary changes.

ANSWER KEY

The following provides the answers and references for the Practice Test questions. Focus Points are referenced using the following abbreviations:
T = Text and V = Video

	Answers	Learning Objectives	Focus Points	References
1.	D	1	T1	Hales, p. 192
2.	B	1	T2	Hales, p. 193
3.	C	1	T3	Hales, p. 197
4.	C	1	T3	Hales, p. 200
5.	C	1	T4	Hales, p. 204
6.	C	2	T5	Hales, pp. 209, 212
7.	D	2	T6	Hales, p. 209
8.	B	1	V1	Video
9.	A	2	V2	Video
10.	C	2	V3	Video
11.	B	1	V4	Video
12.	basal metabolic rate	1	T1	Hales, p. 193
13.	bulimia nervosa	1	T3	Hales, p. 201
14.	cellulite	2	T6	Hales, p. 209
15.	sedentary	1	V1	Video
16.	exercise	2	V3	Video
17.	T	2	V2	Video

Lesson 8

Intimate Relationships

The pure relationship, how beautiful it is! How easily it is damaged, or weighed down with irrelevancies—not even irrelevancies, just life itself, the accumulations of life and of time. For the first part of every relationship is pure, whether it be friend or lover, husband or child. It is pure, simple, and unencumbered. It is like the artist's vision before he has to discipline it into form, or like the flower of love before it has ripened into the firm but heavy fruit of responsibility. Two people listening to each other, two shells meeting each other, making one world between them. There are no others in the perfect unity of that instant, no other people or things or interests. It is free of ties or claims, unburdened by responsibilities, by worry about the future, or debts to the past.

—Anne Morrow Lindbergh, *Gift from the Sea*

LESSON ASSIGNMENT

Review the following assignment in order to schedule your time appropriately. Pay careful attention; the titles and numbers of the textbook chapter, the telecourse guide lesson, and the video program may be different from one another.

Text:

Hales, *An Invitation to Health,*
Chapter 7, "Communication and Relationships," pp. 218–237 and pp. 242–245.
Chapter 17, "Staying Safe: Preventing Injury, Violence, and Victimization," pp. 584–585.

Video:

"Intimate Relationships"
from the series *Living with Health.*

OVERVIEW

Think about the relationships you have had in your life. How many truly intimate relationships have you had? How many people do you know with whom you can share your deepest secrets, your true feelings, and innermost thoughts? How many people share this intimate climate of trust and acceptance with you? Not very many? This is not surprising, though you may be surprised when you actually think about it. We all need this nurturance, acceptance, and trust—in a word, intimacy. Yet it may be difficult to attain and complex to maintain. We first experience intimacy with our parents, then grow to other close relationships with siblings and friends, then develop romantic relationships. For many of us, marriage is the most intimate relationship of all. Throughout our lives we need intimacy, though our relationships with others change as we grow and change. In order to attain intimacy with another, we must have positive self-esteem, self-efficacy, feelings of caring, sharing, trust, commitment, and tenderness toward that person. In other words, we must truly care deeply about that person, whether the person is a best friend or lover. In a good marriage, the partners may be best friends and lovers, but all intimate relationships are by no means sexual ones. Some of the most powerful intimacy is seen in lifelong friends.

Developing an intimate romantic relationship, choosing a mate, making the decision to commit to that person, and sustaining a long-term intimate relationship requires much work, but is worth whatever effort we put into it. Too often, we "fall in love" without much thought or concern about the commitment we must be willing to make to sustain the relationship. That intense romantic love that brings us together can rarely be sustained as the years go by, so we must have the deep trust, sharing, affection, and togetherness that is the companionate love that sustains the long-term relationship or marriage.

Though most people marry, there are other very normal lifestyles such as single living and cohabitation. The same need for intimacy is present in people living in these lifestyles. The cohabiting couple is very similar to the married couple in the characteristics and needs of the intimate relationship. The single person may have more difficulty finding those intimate relationships, but certainly needs intimate friends just as do all of us.

Some of the most dramatic changes in the nature of relationships have come in the form of marriages that end with divorce. In the past the idea of "till death do us part" was taken quite literally. People stayed in unhappy marriages for a variety of reasons, frequently because they felt it was better for the children. People today are much less willing to stay in a relationship if they are not getting along and the relationship is not a happy one. While divorce is difficult for everyone involved, it can be a positive solution to a serious relationship problem.

Far worse than any divorce is the occurrence of violence in a relationship. Domestic violence is an alarming problem that affects all segments of the population. The outbreak of violence or abuse in a relationship signifies major problems that must be dealt with professionally. It is absolutely essential that the victim take action to get out of the situation before the violence moves to tragedy.

Building and sustaining a lasting intimate relationship requires us to first have a sense of our own identity, then to be willing to share, to give and receive love, to communicate effectively, and most of all to truly commit to that person and the relationship.

LEARNING OBJECTIVES

Goal

You should be able to discuss the characteristics and importance of intimate relationships, the importance of communication in relationships, the progression of relationships from friendship to mature love, marriage, and problems that may develop in committed relationships.

Objectives

Upon completion of this lesson, you should be able to:

1. Define friendship. Describe the progression of a relationship from friendship to mature love, including the behavioral expectations of each phase, the importance of communication, and ways to end a relationship.

2. Discuss living arrangement options available to adults, the various types of marriages, and ways to avoid problems, including domestic violence, that many develop.

KEY TERMS

Look for these items as you proceed through the lesson assignments. Be able to discuss them upon completion of this lesson.

intimacy
cohabitation
companion-oriented marriage
rescue marriage
romantic marriage
traditional marriage
enabling

TEXT FOCUS POINTS

The following focus points are designed to help you get the most from the text. Review them, then read the assignment. You may want to write notes to reinforce what you have learned.

Text: Hales, *An Invitation to Health,* Chapter 7, pp. 218–237 and pp. 242–245, and Chapter 17, pp. 584–585.

1. Analyze the role of verbal and nonverbal communication in building a relationship. How do men and women typically differ in communicating?
2. Define friendship and explain how friendship grows.
3. Compare and contrast the behavioral expectations for friendship, dating, and mature love.
4. Describe the typical progress of a relationship from dating to mature love. Define intimacy and explain its role in a relationship.
5. How should one end a relationship? Discuss strategies for dealing with rejection.
6. Explain living arrangement options that today's adults have.
7. Compare the different types of marriages.

8. What are some of the common problems that occur in committed relationships? How can some of these be prevented?

9. Describe the abuse pattern and explain how it relates to partner abuse.

VIDEO FOCUS POINTS

The following focus points are designed to help you get the most from the video segment of this lesson. Review them, then watch the video. You may want to write notes to reinforce what you have learned.

Video: "Intimate Relationships"

1. What are some of the important considerations in selecting a mate? What part do attraction, romance, and love play in a relationship?

2. Discuss characteristics important in intimate relationships.

3. What kinds of things are important in sustaining long-term intimate relationships?

4. How do problems of violence develop in relationships? What can be done to improve these relationships?

INDIVIDUAL HEALTH PLAN

This portion of the lesson is designed to enable you to use the information you have learned in your own life situation to improve the quality of your life. You should do any exercise assigned, complete the journal portion of the plan, then put this portion of the health plan into practice in your life.

> Complete the Self-Survey, "How Strong Is the Communication and Affection in Your Relationship?" on page 229. If you have a partner or significant other, have that person complete the survey. Discuss your responses and make plans to work on areas of need.
>
> In your journal, list those individuals with whom you have a close relationship. Explain why these relationships are special and what each of you brings to the relationship.

RELATED ACTIVITIES

These activities are not required unless your instructor assigns them. They are offered as suggestions to help you learn more about the material presented in this lesson.

1. Interview some of your friends who are married, some who are single, and some who are cohabiting. Ask them about their thoughts on intimacy. Ask them about the characteristics of their relationships, what strengths they have, and what difficulties they encounter.

2. Visit or call an agency that deals with battered spouses and domestic violence. Ask what kinds of issues seem to lead to violence, what are typical outcomes, and other questions that you are interested in.

PRACTICE TEST

After reading the assignment and watching the video, you should be able to answer the Practice Test questions. Tests also include essay questions that are similar to the Text Focus Points and the Video Focus Points. When you have completed the Practice Test questions, turn to the Answer Key to score your answers.

Multiple-Choice

Select the one choice that best answers the question.

1. All of the following might be good strategies to employ to enhance communication EXCEPT __________.
   A. respecting confidences entrusted to you
   B. becoming a better listener
   C. showing interest in the other person by asking about feelings
   D. generalizing statements toward the other person, not yourself

2. All of the following might be good strategies to employ if you wish to maintain good friendships EXCEPT __________.
   A. being very closed and not sharing
   B. being sensitive to friends' feelings
   C. expressing appreciation
   D. talking about your friendship

3. If you were on a game show and had to pick a blind date from a 30-second personal video, which factor, according to statistics, would most likely have the greatest influence on your selection?
   A. Personal appearance
   B. Sexual aura
   C. Expressed opinions
   D. Mutual interests

4. Robert Sternberg defines the triangle of love as that which involves all of the following points EXCEPT __________.
   A. intimacy
   B. passion
   C. infatuation
   D. commitment

5. Which of the following factors would probably have the least influence on your falling in love with another person?
   A. Their values
   B. Their ideas regarding child raising
   C. Their cultural or social backgrounds
   D. Their similarity of interests with yours

6. According to recent research, the main reason both men and women remain single is that they __________.
   A. enjoy their independence
   B. wish to remain more financially stable
   C. haven't found the right person
   D. prefer to focus on their careers

7. All of the following have served to change the traditional view of marriage to the way it is viewed in our society today EXCEPT the __________.
   A. increasing divorce rates
   B. influence of various religions
   C. fewer number of arranged marriages
   D. social acceptance of cohabitation

8. How often should a couple engage in sexual activity to maintain intimacy in their relationship?
   A. At least three times a week
   B. As often as the man desires
   C. As often as is necessary to maintain fertility
   D. As often as is mutually agreeable to each partner

9. Which of the following is probably one of the least reported crimes in the United States?
   A. Arson
   B. Domestic violence
   C. Alcohol-related crime
   D. Drug-related crime

10. Sending flowers and taking the partner out to dinner exemplifies the part of the relationship that is termed __________.
   A. attraction
   B. romance
   C. physical love
   D. companionate love

11. Important requirements for intimacy include all the following EXCEPT _____.
   A. trust
   B. openness
   C. sex
   D. deep caring

12. Most people feel that the one most important factor in sustaining a long-term, intimate relationship is __________.
    A. sexual compatibility
    B. financial agreement
    C. romance
    D. communication

13. The perpetrator of violence in a relationship is usually the one who is more __________.
    A. right
    B. intelligent
    C. powerful
    D. angry

Fill-in-the-Blank

Insert the correct word or words in the blank for each item.

14. ____________ _______ may be based on feelings of elation, desire, and ecstasy.

15. ____________ marriages are where couples assume prescribed societal roles.

16. The two most important factors in a couple's sex life are ____________ and ____________.

17. The initial, positive impression that an individual has of another is termed ______________.

True-False

If the statement is true, write "T" to the left of the statement. If the statement (or any part of the statement) is false, write "F" to the left of the statement.

18. Openness and honesty are important characteristics of successful intimate relationships.

19. Sustaining a successful long-term relationship involves surrendering one's individuality.

ANSWER KEY

The following provides the answers and references for the Practice Test questions. Focus Points are referenced using the following abbreviations:
T = Text and V = Video

	Answers	Learning Objectives	Focus Points	References
1.	D	1	T1	Hales, p. 220
2.	A	1	T2	Hales, p. 224
3.	A	1	T3	Hales, p. 225
4.	C	1	T4	Hales, p. 228
5.	B	1	T5	Hales, pp. 225–226
6.	C	2	T6	Hales, p. 231
7.	B	2	T7	Hales, p. 233
8.	D	2	T8	Hales, p. 235
9.	B	2	T9	Hales, p. 585
10.	B	1	V1	Video
11.	C	1	V2	Video
12.	D	1	V3	Video
13.	C	2	V4	Video
14.	Passionate love	1	T4	Hales, p. 228
15.	Traditional	2	T7	Hales, p. 234
16.	quality and intimacy	2	T7	Hales, p. 235
17.	attraction	1	V1	Video
18.	T	1	V2	Video
19.	F	1	V3	Video

Lesson 9

Sexuality

. . . But it is not only men who have accepted the patriarchal version of reality. Women also have been taught to idealize masculine values at the expense of the feminine side of life. Many women have spent their lives in a constant feeling of inferiority because they felt that to be feminine was "second best." Women have been trained that only masculine activities, thinking, power, and achieving have any real value. Thus Western woman finds herself in the same psychological dilemma as Western man: developing a one-sided, competitive mastery of the masculine qualities at the expense of her feminine side.

—Robert A. Johnson in *We*

LESSON ASSIGNMENT

Review the following assignment in order to schedule your time appropriately. Pay careful attention; the titles and numbers of the textbook chapter, the telecourse guide lesson, and the video program may be different from one another.

Text:

Hales, *An Invitation to Health,*
Chapter 8, "Personal Sexuality," pp. 246–283.
Chapter 17, "Staying Safe: Preventing Injury, Violence, and Victimization," pp. 585–597.

Video:

"Sexuality"
from the series *Living with Health.*

OVERVIEW

Of all the aspects of health, sex and sexuality are probably the most emotionally "charged" and subject to the most myths and misconceptions. We all think about, read about, and are constantly bombarded with messages about sex and sexuality in the media. In spite of this, we frequently are not very sure how we really feel about our own sexuality. Sometimes we even have feelings of guilt about it.

We are all sexual beings. Our gender development begins before we are born. After birth, society places certain expectations on us, depending on our sex. Though our fundamental sense of our maleness or femaleness is set by the time we are about three years old, the expression of our sexuality changes through our life. These expressions of our sexuality make us feel comfortable about ourselves or they can cause tension in our lives. If we have learned to feel comfortable about our sexuality, we will usually feel comfortable with who we are, and be able to enjoy an intimate sexual relationship. If we have learned to feel uncomfortable with our sexuality, we may have considerable difficulty.

Important to a healthy sexuality is an understanding of our sexual anatomy and physiology—in other words, how we work. Here, lack of clear understanding again creates more misconceptions and problems than almost any other aspect of sexuality. For some reason, we often feel more comfortable about any other part of our anatomy and physiology than we do about our sexual selves. If you have not done it already, learn about your sexuality now and enjoy it.

Now is also a good time to also consider the difference in sex and sexuality. Sex, whether we are talking about gender or intercourse, is only a part of sexuality. Our sexuality encompasses who we are, and has even been said to be the "sum total of our personality." Responsible sexual behavior is an important part of that whole picture known as our sexuality. In a caring and supportive intimate relationship, sexual intercourse adds a very special dimension. If the relationship is demeaning or exploitive, the sexual part is also damaging.

Our sexuality is fundamental to our good health. Our decisions about sexual behavior need to help us develop and nurture relationships, rather than hurt or degrade them. If we make responsible decisions, communicate openly, and truly value the relationship, our sexuality will reflect the very best of human intimacy.

LEARNING OBJECTIVES

Goal

You should be able to discuss issues, conditions, and problems of human sexuality; the healthy sexual relationship; the human sexual response; and responsible sexual behavior.

Objectives

Upon completion of this lesson, you should be able to:

1. Explain the major factors that influence sexual identity and gender identity, the sexual relationship, the parts and functions of the male and female reproductive systems, and some of the conditions or issues in women's and in men's health.
2. List and describe the steps in the human sexual response cycle, some of the concerns that people have about sexual performance, and the most effective methods for preventing HIV and other sexually transmitted diseases.
3. Describe the factors that increase the potential for sexual victimization, types of sexual violence, and preventive strategies which decrease the risk of sexual victimization and violence.

KEY TERMS

Look for these items as you proceed through the lesson assignments. Be able to discuss them upon completion of this lesson.

sexuality
sex
intimacy
gender
gonads
hormones
endocrine system
estrogen
progesterone
testosterone
gonadotropins
secondary sex characteristics
androgyny
mons pubis
labia majora
labia minora
clitoris
vagina
perineum
cervix
uterus
endometrium
ovaries
ova (ovum)
fallopian tubes
ovulation
corpus luteum
menstruation
premenstrual syndrome (PMS)
dysmenorrhea
amenorrhea
menopause
hormone replacement therapy (HRT)
penis
scrotum
testes
sperm
epididymis
urethra
semen
vas deferens
seminal vesicles
ejaculatory duct
prostate gland
Cowper's glands
circumcision
prostatitis
benign prostatic hypertrophy
abstinence
nocturnal emissions
masturbation
sexual orientation
celibacy
bisexual
heterosexual
homosexual
erogenous
intercourse
orgasm
cunnilingus
fellatio
ejaculation
refractory period
impotence
premature ejaculation
dyspareunia
vaginismus
sexual compulsion
transgendered
quid pro quo
hostile offensive environment
sexual coercion
rape

TEXT FOCUS POINTS

The following focus points are designed to help you get the most from the text. Review them, then read the assignment. You may want to write notes to reinforce what you have learned.

Text: Hales, *An Invitation to Health*, Chapter 8, pp. 246–283 and Chapter 17, pp. 585–597.

1. Explain the major factors that influence sexual identity and gender identity in our society.

2. Name the parts of the female reproductive system and describe the function of each part. Do the same for the parts of the male reproductive system.

3. What are some conditions or issues unique to women's health? to men's health? Discuss these as well as conditions common to both men and women. Define sexual health and sexually healthy relationships.

4. List and briefly describe each step in the human sexual response cycle. What differences exist between the sexual response cycles of males and females?

5. Describe some methods for preventing infection from HIV and other sexually transmitted diseases.

6. List and explain some of the common concerns of men and women about sexual performance difficulties. What options do these people have for help with these conditions?

7. Define sexual victimization, sexual harassment, and sexual coercion, and explain how each can develop.

8. List the different types of rape and describe recommended actions for preventing rape and sexual violence.

VIDEO FOCUS POINTS

The following focus points are designed to help you get the most from the video segment of this lesson. Review them, then watch the video. You may want to write notes to reinforce what you have learned.

Video: "Sexuality"

1. How have attitudes about sex, sexuality, and gender roles changed in recent years?

2. What role does sex play in a relationship that is nurturing, caring, and sharing?

3. Explain the boundaries between sex that is nurturing and that which is unacceptable and demeaning. Include a discussion of rape as an act of violence.

INDIVIDUAL HEALTH PLAN

This portion of the lesson is designed to enable you to use the information you have learned in your own life situation to improve the quality of your life. You should do any exercise assigned, complete the journal portion of the plan, then put this portion of the health plan into practice in your life.

> Compete the Self-Survey, "How Much Do You Know About Sex?" on p. 260. If you find that you know less about sex than you thought, spend extra time studying this lesson and other material related to it. In your journal, record your feelings about your own sexuality. Does your sexual behavior match your sexual values? Develop your own plan for responsible sexual expression. Be certain these plans fit you and are not what you think someone else expects of you.

RELATED ACTIVITIES

These activities are not required unless your instructor assigns them. They are offered as suggestions to help you learn more about the material presented in this lesson.

1. Interview a sexual therapist to learn more about sexual problems in relationships and their treatment.

2. Discuss the subject of sexuality with some of your close friends of both sexes. Compare and contrast the different ideas.

3. Find out how a rape crisis center operates, some of the problems suffered by rape victims, and some of the legal aspects of a rape investigation.

PRACTICE TEST

After reading the assignment and watching the video, you should be able to answer the Practice Test questions. Tests also include essay questions that are similar to the Text Focus Points and the Video Focus Points. When you have completed the Practice Test questions, turn to the Answer Key to score your answers.

Multiple-Choice

Select the one choice that best answers the question.

1. The combination of an "X" chromosome from the mother and an "X" chromosome from the father results in __________.
   A. a genetic female
   B. a genetic male
   C. none of the above, there is not enough information to determine gender
   D. none of the above, because the father can't supply an "X" chromosome

2. The opening to the womb or the uterus is called the __________.
   A. perineum
   B. cervix
   C. urethra
   D. placenta

3. All of the following may be causes of premenstrual syndrome EXCEPT ______.
   A. hormonal imbalances
   B. stress
   C. sexual celibacy
   D. brain chemical changes

4. Sexual intercourse is called __________.
   A. cunnilingus
   B. fellatio
   C. coitus
   D. vaginitis

5. Which of the following activities would most likely spread the virus that causes AIDS?
   A. Having sexual intercourse with an infected partner while wearing a condom and using a vaginal spermicide
   B. Intimate kissing with a partner whose sexual history you do not know
   C. Donating blood in a large metropolitan area
   D. Sharing needles with a close friend

6. All of the following are true statements regarding male sexual arousal difficulties EXCEPT __________.
   A. men who smoke have higher rates of impotence
   B. impotence has been defined as being unable to achieve and maintain an erection
   C. topical anesthetics used to prevent premature ejaculation in men will dull the pleasure of intercourse for female partners
   D. consistent delaying of orgasm by a man can lead to impotence over time

7. Which of the following is the most accurate statement regarding pornography and sexual victimization?
   A. Men who read pornography are more likely to rape women.
   B. People who read child pornography are also more likely to commit rape.
   C. Men who read violent pornography are less likely to see rape as a crime.
   D. People who don't read pornography don't engage in sexual crimes.

8. A rape committed by multiple attackers on a victim is called a _______ rape.
   A. gang
   B. power
   C. acquaintance
   D. violent

9. A negative aspect of the changing attitudes about sex and sexuality is the _____.
   A. growth of the women's movement
   B. perception of sexuality as a "closet" topic
   C. exploitation of women and sexuality
   D. development of a men's movement

10. In a nurturing relationship, sex __________.
    A. occurs at least once a week
    B. plays a minor role
    C. presents many problems
    D. deepens the relationship

11. During which of the following circumstances is sex always unacceptable?
    A. It is exploitive.
    B. It is not wanted by one partner.
    C. It is demeaning.
    D. All of the above.

Fill-in-the-Blank

Insert the correct word or words in the blank for each item.

12. The two primary female hormones are ____________ and ____________.

13. The surgical removal of the foreskin usually done just after birth is known as ________________.

14. The recovery time men experience during the resolution phase of the sexual cycle after orgasm is known as the ________________ ____________.

15. Coercing a person to engage in sexual intercourse when the person resists is considered ____________.

True-False

If the statement is true, write "T" to the left of the statement. If the statement (or any part of the statement) is false, write "F" to the left of the statement.

16. Attitudes about sex and sexuality have changed little through the years.

17. When a relationship is nurturing and caring, sex plays only a minor role.

18. The psychological effects of rape on the victim begin with extreme fear and extend to long-term feelings of lack of control and questioning oneself.

ANSWER KEY

The following provides the answers and references for the Practice Test questions. Focus Points are referenced using the following abbreviations:

T = Text and V = Video

	Answers	Learning Objectives	Focus Points	References
1.	A	1	T1	Hales, p. 248
2.	B	1	T2	Hales, p. 251
3.	C	1	T3	Hales, p. 253
4.	C	2	T4	Hales, p. 271
5.	D	2	T5	Hales, p. 398
6.	D	2	T6	Hales, pp. 276–277
7.	C	3	T7	Hales, p. 280
8.	A	3	T8	Hales, p. 589
9.	C	1	V1	Video
10.	D	1	V2	Video
11.	D	3	V3	Video
12.	estrogen/progesterone	1	T2	Hales, p. 248
13.	circumcision	1	T3	Hales, p. 257
14.	refractory period	2	T4	Hales, p. 275
15.	rape	3	V3	Video
16.	F	1	V1	Video
17.	F	1	V2	Video
18.	T	3	V3	Video

Lesson 10

Reproduction and Sexual Health

Birth is a metaphor for life. How we plan for it, how we experience it, how we feel about it afterward are all part of who we are.
—Rahima Baldwin and Terra Palmarini, *Pregnant Feelings*

LESSON ASSIGNMENT

Review the following assignment in order to schedule your time appropriately. Pay careful attention; the titles and numbers of the textbook chapter, the telecourse guide lesson, and the video program may be different from one another.

Text:

Hales, *An Invitation to Health,*
Chapter 9, "Reproductive Choices," pp. 284–330.

Video:

"Reproduction and Sexual Health"
from the series *Living with Health.*

OVERVIEW

Many of us think of sexual intercourse as simply a part of an intimate relationship and give little thought to its role in beginning a new life. Thus, sexual intercourse is intertwined with the most significant decision that we will ever make—the decision to have children. Never before in history have there ever been so many issues involving sexual health. For this reason, this lesson is particularly important. The decisions you make about your sexual activity will greatly influence your overall health.

Having intercourse without understanding the anatomy and physiology of reproduction, birth control options, and the process of pregnancy can be compared to taking a very hot sports car for a spin without learning to drive. Lack of knowledge and sexual irresponsibility frequently result in sexually transmitted diseases, problem pregnancies, unwanted children, and child abuse. Knowledge, understanding, and responsible behavior result in mature, caring relationships and nurtured children. There are also differing values concerning birth control. The important thing to consider is that sexual intercourse without some form of birth control amounts to a decision to have children.

There is nothing more remarkable than the growth of a single cell into a perfectly formed human infant. When you consider how many things can happen in the process of conception, the development of the embryo into a fetus, and the growth of the fetus during pregnancy, the remarkable becomes a true miracle. In spite of incredible progress in medicine and technology in treating problems of the fetus and newborn, the United States has a staggering number of infants suffering from the effects of parental substance abuse and other preventable problems. These babies are really the ones who are suffering for their parents' neglect and abuse. Pregnancy is probably the most important time of life to practice a healthy lifestyle, not only for oneself, but for the precious life that is to come.

If you have or plan to have a sexual relationship, it is imperative that you examine your sexual health behavior and values. This lesson is not about telling you what to think about birth control, abortion, and other sexual issues. It is about encouraging you to think and make responsible sexual health decisions based on your own knowledge and values.

LEARNING OBJECTIVES

Goal

You should be able to explain conception, the reproductive process, contraception, pregnancy, and childbirth.

Objectives

Upon completion of this lesson, you should be able to:

1. Explain conception, the physiology of pregnancy, fetal development, labor and delivery, and options for infertile couples.

2. Discuss the major options for contraception, the issues of abortion, and the implications of unhealthy lifestyles on the fetus.

KEY TERMS

Look for these items as you proceed through the lesson assignments. Be able to discuss them upon completion of this lesson.

conception
spermatogenesis
fertilization
zygote
implantation
contraception
failure rate
coitus interruptus
oral contraceptives
constant-dose combination pill
multiphasic pill
progestin-only pill
minipill
barrier contraceptives
condom
diaphragm
cervical cap
vaginal spermicides
vaginal contraceptive film (VCF)
intrauterine device (IUD)
sterilization
vasectomy
tubal ligation
laparotomy
laparoscopy
colpotomy
hysterectomy
ovulation method
rhythm method
basal body temperature
after-intercourse methods
elective abortion
suction curettage
dilation and evacuation (D&E)
hysterotomy
preconception care
amnion
embryo
fetus
placenta
fetal alcohol syndrome (FAS)
perinatology
ectopic pregnancy
miscarriage
rubella
premature labor
psychoprophylaxis
Lamaze method
epidural block
spinal block
labor
breech birth
caesarean delivery
postpartum depression
lochia
sudden infant death syndrome (SIDS)
infertility
artificial insemination
adoption

TEXT FOCUS POINTS

The following focus points are designed to help you get the most from the text. Review them, then read the assignment. You may want to write notes to reinforce what you have learned.

Text: Hales, *An Invitation to Health*, Chapter 9, pp. 284–330.

1. Explain the process of conception in humans. What is preconception care? Give some examples.

2. List the major options available for contraception and compare the advantages and risks of each.

3. Define abortion and describe the commonly used abortion methods. Discuss the political aspects of the abortion controversy.

4. Describe the physiological effects of pregnancy on a woman. Include a discussion of the most frequent complications of pregnancy.

5. Trace the growth and development of a fetus from embryo to newborn infant.

6. Explain the stages of labor and birth. Include a discussion of birthing options available.

7. What options are available to infertile couples wishing to become parents?

VIDEO FOCUS POINTS

The following focus points are designed to help you get the most from the video segment of this lesson. Review them, then watch the video. You may want to write notes to reinforce what you have learned.

Video: "Reproduction and Sexual Health"

1. How does the mother maintain health for herself and the developing child through pregnancy?

2. Describe the development of the fetus through the three trimesters of pregnancy. Include the changes taking place in the mother.

3. Describe the process of birth.

4. How do unhealthy lifestyle behaviors of the mother, such as drug abuse, affect the developing child?

INDIVIDUAL HEALTH PLAN

This portion of the lesson is designed to enable you to use the information you have learned in your own life situation to improve the quality of your life. You should do any exercise assigned, complete the journal portion of the plan, then put this portion of the health plan into practice in your life.

> Complete the Self-Survey, "Which Contraceptive Method Is Best for You?" on p. 292. In your journal, list factors that make you ready/unready to have a child at this time. If you are not ready to have a child, are your behaviors supporting this? If not, what do you need to change?

RELATED ACTIVITIES

These activities are not required unless your instructor assigns them. They are offered as suggestions to help you learn more about the material presented in this lesson.

1. Research the current abortion issues from the various points of view.

2. Visit the various types of childbirth facilities in your community. Compare and contrast them in terms of safety, competency of staff, comfort, and support for parents and baby.

PRACTICE TEST

After reading the assignment and watching the video, you should be able to answer the Practice Test questions. Tests also include essay questions that are similar to the Text Focus Points and the Video Focus Points. When you have completed the Practice Test questions, turn to the Answer Key to score your answers.

Multiple-Choice

Select the one choice that best answers the question.

1. Storage of sperm prior to ejaculation occurs in the __________.
   A. vas deferens
   B. epididymis
   C. testes
   D. seminiferous tubules

2. Which of the following methods of birth control would be considered the MOST effective based on failure rates?
   A. Rhythm method
   B. Diaphragm with spermicide
   C. Condom with spermicide
   D. Norplant system

3. MOST estrogen-based forms of oral contraception are a health concern because of the association between estrogen and __________.
   A. colon disease
   B. osteoporosis
   C. breast cancer
   D. none of the above

4. All of the following are potentially true statements regarding male vasectomy EXCEPT __________.
   A. it requires hospitalization for twenty-four hours after completion of procedure
   B. the vas deferens are cut and tied off
   C. infertility is not necessarily immediate
   D. no long-term health effects have been positively associated with this

5. The abortion pill currently being tested for effectiveness in the United States is known as __________.
   A. misoprostol
   B. testosterone enanthate
   C. luteinizing hormone
   D. human chorionic gonadotropin

6. All of the following might be good strategies to follow during pregnancy EXCEPT __________.
   A. taking a daily vitamin tablet with folic acid
   B. continuing to use salt lightly unless salt intake is restricted by a physician
   C. going on a very low calorie diet to restrict weight gain
   D. drinking six to eight glasses of liquids each day

7. Which of the following activities characteristically occurs in the first phase of labor?
   A. Effacement and dilation of the cervix
   B. Delivery of the fetus through the birth canal
   C. Delivery of afterbirth
   D. Release of colostrum

8. All of the following are potential treatments couples may pursue for infertility EXCEPT __________.
   A. in vitro fertilization
   B. gamete intrafallopian transfer
   C. balloon tuboplasty
   D. caesarean delivery

9. Healthy lifestyle behaviors for the pregnant woman do NOT include ________.
   A. balanced diet
   B. regular exercise
   C. occasional glasses of wine
   D. multivitamins

10. During the second trimester of pregnancy, the fetus __________.
    A. develops its heart
    B. grows significantly in length
    C. gains MOST of its weight
    D. remains unrecognizable

11. During the first stage of labor, the cervix __________.
    A. dilates
    B. contracts
    C. remains the same
    D. closes

12. When the mother uses drugs during pregnancy, the baby is __________.
    A. born overweight
    B. born addicted
    C. generally unaffected
    D. stillborn

Fill-in-the-Blank

Insert the correct word or words in the blank for each item.

13. The process by which a woman releases a fertile ovum on a regular cycle is referred to as the process of __________.

14. Contraceptives that function by preventing fertilization by means of blocking the sperm from meeting the egg are referred to as __________ contraceptives.

15. Babies born prior to their predicted arrival date are said to be __________.

16. The pregnancy is divided into thirds, each period called a ______________.

True-False

If the statement is true, write "T" to the left of the statement. If the statement (or any part of the statement) is false, write "F" to the left of the statement.

17. Because of danger to the developing fetus, exercise is discouraged for the pregnant woman.

18. Effects of drug abuse by the mother affect the baby in very dangerous ways.

ANSWER KEY

The following provides the answers and references for the Practice Test questions. Focus Points are referenced using the following abbreviations:

T = Text and V = Video

	Answers	Learning Objectives	Focus Points	References
1.	B	1	T1	Hales, p. 256
2.	D	2	T2	Hales, p. 289
3.	D	2	T2	Hales, p. 293
4.	A	2	T2	Hales, p. 307
5.	A	2	T3	Hales, p. 309
6.	C	1	T4	Hales, p. 315
7.	A	1	T6	Hales, p. 320
8.	D	1	T7	Hales, p. 325
9.	C	1	V1	Video
10.	B	1	V2	Video
11.	A	1	V3	Video
12.	B	2	V4	Video
13.	ovulation	1	T1	Hales, p. 252
14.	barrier	2	T2	Hales, p. 299
15.	premature	1	T5	Hales, p. 319
16.	trimester	1	V2	Video
17.	F	1	V1	Video
18.	T	2	V4	Video

Lesson 11

Parenting

There are only two lasting bequests that we can hope to give our children. One of these is roots; the other, wings.

—Hodding Carter

LESSON ASSIGNMENT

Review the following assignment in order to schedule your time appropriately. Pay careful attention; the titles and numbers of the textbook chapter, the telecourse guide lesson, and the video program may be different from one another.

Text:

Hales, *An Invitation to Health*,
Chapter 7, "Communication and Relationships," pp. 237–245.
Chapter 17, "Staying Safe: Preventing Injury, Violence, and Victimization," pp. 584–585 and pp. 593–594.

Video:

"Parenting"
from the series *Living with Health.*

OVERVIEW

Though many people think of marriage as the greatest commitment that we make in our lives, it is not. Parenthood is that supreme commitment. Children are forever. We may divorce our spouse, but we do not divorce our children. Many of us envision that darling little baby enriching our lives (and they certainly do), but give less thought to the responsibility that we take on when we become parents. The decision to become a parent means that we will protect, nurture, feed, clothe, shelter, and love that child 24 hours a day, 365 days a year. We never stop being parents. For most of us, it is a joyful responsibility, although a big responsibility. Because of this, it is important that we are ready to take responsibility for children, so we must make clear decisions about our sexual behavior. If we have made these decisions and have realistic expectations of parenthood, we are ready to cope with the difficulties and to enjoy the unique experiences we share with our children.

While we have impact on our children's lives in many ways, the primary influence we have is on their health at birth and throughout their growth and development. As the dimensions of health are important to us, they are important to our children. Our parenting has a significant effect on our children's physical, emotional, intellectual, social, and spiritual development. Planning for this begins before the child is conceived, and continues on. Responsibility for insuring that the child has a lifestyle that develops the dimensions cannot be ignored or delegated. It belongs to us as parents.

Unfortunately, the antithesis of the healthy functioning family has become a very real problem in America today. Family violence and child abuse are at epidemic proportions. Reasons for this are many, but a common thread is stress within the family. In our roles as individuals, spouses, and parents, we will experience stress. It is important to the well-being of our children and ourselves, that we learn healthy ways of coping and parenting. It is up to us to make certain that our children are not raised in an atmosphere of violence.

While all of this may sound very one-sided, we get much from our children. It has been said that children are our mirror, and this is at least partially true. Children respond and flourish with good parenting. They give us a sense of accomplishment and purpose, and enrich the quality of our life immensely. For all the difficulties and demands, most parents cherish the experience above all else.

LEARNING OBJECTIVES

Goal

You should be able to explain the role and responsibilities of parenthood in the healthy growth and development of the child.

Objectives

Upon completion of this lesson, you should be able to:

1. Describe the changes occurring in family structure, and explain the issues and needs involved in parenting.
2. Discuss the problems of child abuse.

KEY TERMS

Look for these items as you proceed through the lesson assignments. Be able to discuss them upon completion of this lesson.

family
blended family
codependence
dysfunctional
pedophilia
incest

TEXT FOCUS POINTS

The following focus points are designed to help you get the most from the text. Review them, then read the assignment. You may want to write notes to reinforce what you have learned.

Text: Hales, *An Invitation to Health*, Chapter Chapter 7, pp. 237–245 and Chapter 17, pp. 584–585 and pp. 593–594.

1. How has the structure of the family changed through the years?
2. Name and discuss some of the major issues facing parents today.
3. What types of needs do children have?
4. What are some of the causes for dysfunctional relationships? How can some of these be solved?

VIDEO FOCUS POINTS

The following focus points are designed to help you get the most from the video segment of this lesson. Review them, then watch the video. You may want to write notes to reinforce what you have learned.

Video: "Parenting"

1. In what ways has the role of parenthood changed through recent years?

2. Explain the ways in which parents help their children grow in the dimensions, which include physical, emotional, intellectual, social, and spiritual.

3. Describe some of the special challenges that are faced by single parents.

4. Discuss the scope of child abuse in the United States, the effects of abuse on children's health, and things that lower the risk of child abuse.

INDIVIDUAL HEALTH PLAN

This portion of the lesson is designed to enable you to use the information you have learned in your own life situation to improve the quality of your life. You should do any exercise assigned, complete the journal portion of the plan, then put this portion of the health plan into practice in your life.

> In your journal, make a list of your own reasons for having and for not having a child at this time. (Do this even if you have children.) Also list the adjustments you would have to make in your life if you did have a child at this time. Include child-care planning if both parents work or if yours is a single-parent family. How would you adjust your budget to accommodate a child? Write a synopsis of what you found. Are you ready??

RELATED ACTIVITIES

These activities are not required unless your instructor assigns them. They are offered as suggestions to help you learn more about the material presented in this lesson.

1. If you do not have children, interview the parents of children of various ages, concerning the positive experiences and difficulties of parenting.

2. Visit different types of child-care facilities. Find out about their programs, costs, licensing, etc.

PRACTICE TEST

After reading the assignment and watching the video, you should be able to answer the Practice Test questions. Tests also include essay questions that are similar to the Text Focus Points and the Video Focus Points. When you have completed the Practice Test questions, turn to the Answer Key to score your answers.

Multiple-Choice

Select the one choice that best answers the question.

1. The structure of the family has changed through the years in the following ways EXCEPT __________.
   A. marriages are dissolving more often
   B. in many countries, divorce rates doubled between 1970 and 1990
   C. the number of single-parent families is declining
   D. single-parent households are likely to be poorer

2. Which of the following has been shown to be the greatest predictor of marital jeopardy when a baby arrives?
   A. Infrequent sex
   B. A couple's decision not to have children
   C. An extramarital affair
   D. Husband's dissatisfaction with the relationship

3. The child's greatest need is __________.
   A. financial security
   B. love
   C. confidence
   D. high-quality nourishment

4. All of the following might be good strategies to employ to help children adjust to divorce EXCEPT __________.
   A. letting children know there is no bad parent in the divorce
   B. spending extra time with children to help them communicate feelings
   C. letting children know they aren't responsible for the breakup
   D. giving children toys after the divorce to divert their focus from the breakup

5. All of the following are considered components of enabling (codependent) behavior EXCEPT __________.
   A. shielding—covering up for an abuser
   B. controlling—attempting to control another's behavior
   C. rescuing—overprotecting to the point of allowing addictive behavior
   D. guiding—insisting on getting an addict some professional help

6. Changes in the parenting role through the years do NOT include an increase in __________.
   A. single parents
   B. the importance of nurturing
   C. involvement of fathers
   D. child abuse

7. The most critical years in the development of the child are from birth to _______.
   A. five years
   B. ten years
   C. twelve years
   D. eighteen years

8. The single parent most often feels the pressure of __________.
   A. having too little money
   B. being alone in caring for the child
   C. feeling loneliness for the spouse
   D. not wanting the child

9. Child abuse occurs among __________.
   A. lower socioeconomic groups only
   B. all segments of society
   C. mostly single parents
   D. some ethnic groups more than others

Fill-in-the-Blank

Insert the correct word or words in the blank for each item.

10. The years of transition from childhood to adulthood are known as the ______________ years.

11. A family composed of individuals from two separate families is known as a ___________ family.

12. The most difficult form of child abuse to recognize is ___________________.

True-False

If the statement is true, write "T" to the left of the statement. If the statement (or any part of the statement) is false, write "F" to the left of the statement.

13. Joblessness, divorce, and poverty place great pressure on parents but are of little concern to children.

14. Children of single parents usually receive less nurturing than those in two-parent homes.

15. Support systems such as grandparents and other relatives decrease the risk for child abuse.

ANSWER KEY

The following provides the answers and references for the Practice Test questions. Focus Points are referenced using the following abbreviations:
T = Text and V = Video

	Answers	Learning Objectives	Focus Points	References
1.	C	1	T1	Hales, p. 239
2.	D	1	T1	Hales, p. 238
3.	B	1	T3	Hales, p. 238
4.	D	1	T2	Hales, p. 240
5.	D	1	T4	Hales, pp. 241–242
6.	B	1	V1	Video
7.	A	1	V2	Video
8.	B	1	V3	Video
9.	B	2	V4	Video
10.	teen/teenage	1	T2	Hales, p. 239
11.	blended	1	T1	Hales, p. 240
12.	emotional	2	V4	Video
13.	F	1	V1	Video
14.	F	1	V3	Video
15.	T	2	V4	Video

Lesson 12

Communicable Diseases

. . . I think the nuts and bolts that we have, the vaccines, the antibiotics, and the public health measures that limit exposure; that's where we're going to control the infectious disease.

—John Bartlett, M.D.

LESSON ASSIGNMENT

Review the following assignment in order to schedule your time appropriately. Pay careful attention; the titles and numbers of the textbook chapter, the telecourse guide lesson, and the video program may be different from one another.

Text:

Hales, *An Invitation to Health,*
Chapter 11, "Protecting Yourself from Infectious Diseases," pp. 364–384 and pp. 403–407.

Video:

"Communicable Diseases"
from the series *Living with Health.*

OVERVIEW

Disease has been a part of our lives since the dawn of history. Though the causes of many of the great epidemics of the past have been eradicated or brought under control, new diseases are constantly appearing: Lyme disease, HIV/AIDS. Old diseases thought to be under control reappear as threats when conditions change: tuberculosis. Some seem to have always been with us: colds, flu. Our lifestyle, travel, and the progress of medical science all have had a part in changing the patterns of the diseases that threaten us. Clearly the only constant is that, though their appearance may change, diseases remain a part of our lives now and probably will in the foreseeable future.

Because we will be studying various types of disease throughout this course, it is important to understand the different classifications: acute, chronic, infectious, noninfectious, communicable, and noncommunicable. This lesson focuses on the infectious, communicable diseases. To use a simple term, these are diseases that you can "catch." The significance of these communicable diseases is seen many times through history. The "Black Plague" ravaged Europe in the Middle Ages. Groups of native people were wiped out by diseases caught from explorers. Extreme caution was taken by NASA scientists on the first landing on the moon to insure that we did not infect that environment with our organisms and that the mission did not bring any foreign organisms back to earth.

There are several useful models that scientists use to explain how people contract disease. One, the agent-host-environment model, demonstrates the multiplicity of factors that are involved in the onset of disease in the individual. The keys are in the interrelationships of the agent (disease-causing organisms), the host (characteristics of individuals that make them susceptible to the disease), and the environment (extrinsic biological, social, and physical factors that influence the probability of developing an infection).

It is important for us to understand the agents of infection, the ways in which our bodies fight infection, and ways to enhance our resistance to disease. If we practice good health habits based on an understanding of these principles, we will certainly add to our overall health and well-being.

LEARNING OBJECTIVES

Goal

You should be able to explain the infection process, including the agents of infection, be able to compare the various vectors and the ways in which the body defends itself against infectious disease, and describe the most common infectious diseases.

Objectives

Upon completion of this lesson, you should be able to:

1. Explain the infection process, describe the agents of infection, and compare the means of transmission or vectors.
2. List and describe some of the common infectious diseases and analyze the ways in which the body is protected against disease, including immunization.

KEY TERMS

Look for these items as you proceed through the lesson assignments. Be able to discuss them upon completion of this lesson.

pathogen
host
vector
virus
antibiotics
antiviral drug
bacteria
fungi
protozoa
helminth
incubation period
immunity
humoral
gamma globulin
cell-mediated
lymph nodes
inflammation
abscess
systemic disease
allergy
immunotherapy
autoimmune
immune deficiency
influenza
mononucleosis
chronic fatigue syndrome (CFS)
hepatitis
pneumonia
tuberculosis
toxic shock syndrome (TSS)
Lyme disease
trichomoniasis
candidiasis
bacterial vaginosis
pyelonephritis

TEXT FOCUS POINTS

The following focus points are designed to help you get the most from the text. Review them, then read the assignment. You may want to write notes to reinforce what you have learned.

Text: Hales, *An Invitation to Health,* Chapter 11, pp. 364–384 and pp. 403–407.

1. Explain the infection process and describe the different agents of infection.

2. Compare the various means of transmission or vectors.

3. Describe how the body protects itself from infectious disease. Include the role and importance of immunization.

4. List and describe some of the common infectious diseases. Include preventive measures that are effective in protecting the individual from diseases.

VIDEO FOCUS POINTS

The following focus points are designed to help you get the most from the video segment of this lesson. Review them, then watch the video. You may want to write notes to reinforce what you have learned.

Video: "Communicable Diseases"

1. How does the agent-host-environment model explain the spread of communicable disease?

2. How does infectious/communicable disease differ from other forms of disease?

3. How do changes in lifestyles, social conditions, and other factors change the incidence of and potential for communicable disease?

4. Describe the three lines of defense the body has against communicable disease.

5. What control does the individual have over communicable disease?

INDIVIDUAL HEALTH PLAN

This portion of the lesson is designed to enable you to use the information you have learned in your own life situation to improve the quality of your life. You should do any exercise assigned, complete the journal portion of the plan, then put this portion of the health plan into practice in your life.

> In your journal, list the illnesses you have had during the past year. How many of these were infectious? If you know how you contracted them, describe this. Who else in your family had the illness? How might you have protected yourself against the illness?

RELATED ACTIVITIES

These activities are not required unless your instructor assigns them. They are offered as suggestions to help you learn more about the material presented in this lesson.

1. Explore the resurgence of tuberculosis as a public health threat by interviewing a health professional who works with patients who have the disease.

2. Interview a pediatric health professional and ask about the importance of childhood immunization.

3. Discuss with a health department official measures being taken in your community to prevent the spread of disease.

PRACTICE TEST

After reading the assignment and watching the video, you should be able to answer the Practice Test questions. Tests also include essay questions that are similar to the Text Focus Points and the Video Focus Points. When you have completed the Practice Test questions, turn to the Answer Key to score your answers.

Multiple-Choice

Select the one choice that best answers the question.

1. The toughest pathogens for the human body to combat are __________.
   A. bacteria
   B. viruses
   C. protozoa
   D. fungi

2. All of the following are common diseases caused by viruses EXCEPT ______.
   A. influenza
   B. herpes simplex
   C. hepatitis
   D. tuberculosis

3. All of the following diseases are primarily foodborne EXCEPT __________.
   A. salmonella
   B. tuberculosis
   C. botulism
   D. escherichia coli

4. If you are unsure of your past immunizations, a blood test can indicate whether you carry specific __________.
   A. antibodies
   B. weakened antigens
   C. gamma globulin
   D. lymphocytes

5. The leading cause of infectious disease in the United States annually is _______.
   A. tetanus
   B. AIDS
   C. pneumonia and influenza
   D. smallpox

6. All of the following are true statements regarding urinary tract infections EXCEPT __________.
   A. most people who get them have recurrent infections
   B. more women get these than men
   C. they are usually viral in nature
   D. the greatest danger from these is to the kidneys

7. General health of the individual which contributes to vulnerability to a disease like tuberculosis is a condition of the __________.
   A. environment
   B. host
   C. agent
   D. bacteria

8. Communicable diseases are caused by all the following EXCEPT __________.
   A. bacteria
   B. carcinogens
   C. viruses
   D. fungi

9. The body's three lines of defense against disease include all the following EXCEPT __________.
   A. antibiotics
   B. skin and mucus membranes
   C. immunity
   D. inflammatory response

Fill-in-the-Blank

Insert the correct word or words in the blank for each item.

10. Drugs that are used to contain viral infections are known as ____________ drugs.

11. The failure of the body to recognize its own body tissue and therefore attack its own body tissue as an invader is known as ______________ disorder.

12. Urinary tract infections that attack the kidneys are known as ________________.

13. Health habits that increase the potential for disease are factors relating to the ________________.

14. The outside means by which the body's immunity can be increased is termed ____________________.

True-False

If the statement is true, write "T" to the left of the statement. If the statement (or any part of the statement) is false, write "F" to the left of the statement.

15. Tuberculosis is a good example of a disease that has had a recurrence because of changes in factors related to the agent, hosts, and environments.

16. In contrast to many other diseases, the individual has very little control over the spread of communicable disease.

ANSWER KEY

The following provides the answers and references for the Practice Test questions. Focus Points are referenced using the following abbreviations:

T = Text and V = Video

	Answers	Learning Objectives	Focus Points	References
1.	B	1	T1	Hales, p. 366
2.	D	1	T1	Hales, p. 367
3.	B	1	T2	Hales, p. 367
4.	A	2	T3	Hales, p. 373
5.	C	2	T4	Hales, p. 380
6.	C	2	T4	Hales, p. 384
7.	B	1	V1	Video
8.	B	1	V2	Video
9.	A	2	V4	Video
10.	antiviral	1	T1	Hales, p. 367
11.	autoimmune	2	T3	Hales, p. 372
12.	pyelonephritis	2	T4	Hales, p. 384
13.	host	1	V1	Video
14.	immunization	2	V4	Video
15.	T	1	V3	Video
16.	F	2	V5	Video

Lesson 13

AIDS and Sexually Transmitted Diseases

America is in great danger—not of catching AIDS—but of losing its humanity. . . . In all history there has never been a cure for that.

—Belinda Mason

LESSON ASSIGNMENT

Review the following assignment in order to schedule your time appropriately. Pay careful attention; the titles and numbers of the textbook chapter, the telecourse guide lesson, and the video program may be different from one another.

Text:

Hales, *An Invitation to Health*,
Chapter 11, "Protecting Yourself from Infectious Diseases," pp. 384–407.

Video:

"AIDS and Sexually Transmitted Diseases"
from the series *Living with Health*.

OVERVIEW

While most of the communicable diseases are on the decline, or at least under control, incidence of sexually transmitted diseases is rising at an alarming rate. The reasons for this increase are many. The most important step in the solution—prevention—is the responsibility of all of us.

Though HIV/AIDS is receiving most of the attention at the present time, large numbers of people are being infected with the other sexually transmitted diseases (STDs), most of which have been around for a long time. We all know the severity of HIV/AIDS, but many of us overlook the severe and lasting effects the other STDs can have, such as sterility, abnormal pregnancy, and increased risk of cancer. Most STDs are caused by bacteria or viruses. Those caused by bacteria can usually be cured with antibiotics. Those caused by viruses cannot be cured because we have no cure for viral infections. Treatment is aimed at controlling the symptoms and preventing the spread of the disease to other people.

HIV/AIDS has received great attention, and those who have it are frequently ostracized and degraded. The truth is that AIDS is a disease, and the people who have it are entitled to our care and concern, just as those with any serious disease. Once thought to be a disease confined to homosexual men and intravenous drug users, now HIV/AIDS is understood to be a threat to others. Today, heterosexual people in developing countries have the highest incidence of HIV/AIDS. We also know that the risk increases with the number of sexual partners. Because AIDS is a killer disease, with no cure at this time, prevention is the only certain answer.

While a few are exposed to HIV/AIDS and other sexually transmitted diseases through no action of their own, most are spread through unprotected sexual intercourse, and in the case of HIV, through the use of contaminated needles in intravenous drug use. This fact leads us back to the concept of gaining knowledge and being responsible for our own health behavior. The only completely "safe" sex is abstinence. Other than abstinence, using condoms and keeping to a monogamous relationship with a noninfected partner are the preventive measures we can take. In the case of HIV, avoidance of exposure with contaminated intravenous drug paraphernalia is critical.

Knowledge and understanding are crucial to the ultimate control of HIV/AIDS and other sexually transmitted diseases. We must be a part of the solution to the elimination of these diseases, rather than being part of the problem. Most important of all, we must take an active role in the prevention of the disease through our own responsible sexual behavior.

LEARNING OBJECTIVES

Goal

The student should be able to explain HIV/AIDS and other sexually transmitted diseases and to describe responsible sexual behavior that prevents the spread of sexually transmitted diseases.

Objectives

Upon completion of this lesson, you should be able to:

1. Describe the various sexually transmitted diseases including HIV/AIDS, the patterns, their risks, symptoms, treatment, preventive measures, and implications for the future.

2. Discuss the impact of HIV/AIDS on the lives of the patient and family members.

KEY TERMS

sexually transmitted diseases
chlamydial infection
pelvic inflammatory disease (PID)
gonorrhea
nongonococcal urethritis (NGU)
syphilis
herpes simplex
human papilloma virus
chancroid
human immunodeficiency virus (HIV)
acquired immunodeficiency syndrome (AIDS)

TEXT FOCUS POINTS

The following focus points are designed to help you get the most from the text. Review them, then read the assignment. You may want to write notes to reinforce what you have learned.

Text: Hales, *An Invitation to Health*, Chapter 11, pp. 384–407.

1. List and describe the most prevalent sexually transmitted diseases, their symptoms, and treatment.

2. Define HIV infection, including the methods of HIV transmission. Describe the symptoms of HIV infection, and the progression of HIV infection to AIDS.

3. Explain some methods for preventing HIV infection and other sexually transmitted diseases.

VIDEO FOCUS POINTS

The following focus points are designed to help you get the most from the video segment of this lesson. Review them, then watch the video. You may want to write notes to reinforce what you have learned.

Video: "AIDS and Sexually Transmitted Diseases"

1. How widespread and of what significance is the problem of HIV, AIDS, and other sexually transmitted diseases?
2. List the most common sexually transmitted diseases other than HIV and AIDS, and discuss each one, including prevention.
3. Identify the primary modes of transmission of HIV. Describe the impact on the patient and family and discuss prevention.

INDIVIDUAL HEALTH PLAN

This portion of the lesson is designed to enable you to use the information you have learned in your own life situation to improve the quality of your life. You should do any exercise assigned, complete the journal portion of the plan, then put this portion of the health plan into practice in your life.

> Complete the Self-Survey, "STD Attitude Scale," on pages 389–390 of your textbook. In your journal, describe what you have learned about yourself from this exercise. Are there changes you will make in your attitude or in your behavior?

RELATED ACTIVITIES

These activities are not required unless your instructor assigns them. They are offered as suggestions to help you learn more about the material presented in this lesson.

1. Interview someone who works in an AIDS treatment or counseling center and find out what problems HIV/AIDS patients face.

2. Consider serving as a volunteer in some agency that serves HIV/AIDS patients.

PRACTICE TEST

After reading the assignment and watching the video, you should be able to answer the Practice Test questions. Tests also include essay questions that are similar to the Text Focus Points and the Video Focus Points. When you have completed the Practice Test questions, turn to the Answer Key to score your answers.

Multiple-Choice

Select the one choice that best answers the question.

1. If untreated, what disease frequently leads to pelvic inflammatory disease, a painful condition that can cause sterility?
   A. Syphilis
   B. Condyloma
   C. Gonorrhea
   D. Herpes

2. Syphilis is caused by a corkscrew-shaped spiral bacterium called a __________.
   A. staphyloccus
   B. spirochete
   C. condyloma
   D. trichomonas

3. Herpes is NOT __________.
   A. associated with cancer of the cervix
   B. threatening to the unborn child
   C. prevalent throughout the United States
   D. responsive to antibiotics

4. HIV is spread through the following means EXCEPT __________.
   A. airborne transmission
   B. sexual intercourse
   C. contaminated drug equipment
   D. before birth through circulation

5. In many cases, the initial symptoms of HIV infection resemble those of _______.
   A. herpes
   B. cancer
   C. mononucleosis
   D. condyloma

6. Precautions for preventing the spread of HIV/AIDS do NOT include _________.
   A. limiting the number of sexual partners
   B. using condoms during sexual activity
   C. avoiding drug use, particularly intravenous injections
   D. assuming that there is no threat

7. AIDS is described as the most severe form of __________.
   A. cancer
   B. HIV infection
   C. yeast infection
   D. syphilis

8. One of the most disturbing things about AIDS is that it __________.
   A. presents a problem in the United States
   B. affects primarily target groups
   C. exists as a global problem
   D. occurs primarily in third world countries

9. A common viral, sexually transmitted disease that causes blisterlike sores around the genitalia and is very dangerous to the infant at birth is __________.
   A. gonorrhea
   B. genital herpes
   C. chlamydia
   D. HIV

10. Prevention of AIDS includes all the following EXCEPT __________.
    A. using condoms
    B. avoiding IV drug use
    C. taking preventive medication
    D. limiting sexual partners

Fill-in-the-Blank

Insert the correct word or words in the blank for each item.

11. Any inflammation of the urethra that is not of gonorrhea origin is usually generally referred to as ______________ ______________.

12. The very commonly diagnosed sexually transmitted disease characterized by warts in the genital area is known as genital warts or ____________________.

True-False

If the statement is true, write "T" to the left of the statement. If the statement (or any part of the statement) is false, write "F" to the left of the statement.

13. AIDS is the only really serious, sexually transmitted disease.

14. Chlamydia is a widely occurring, sexually transmitted disease affecting only women.

15. Virtually everyone is affected in one way or another by the spread of AIDS.

ANSWER KEY

The following provides the answers and references for the Practice Test questions. Focus Points are referenced using the following abbreviations:

T = Text and V = Video

	Answers	Learning Objectives	Focus Points	References
1.	C	1	T1	Hales, p. 392
2.	B	1	T1	Hales, pp. 387
3.	D	1	T1	Hales, pp. 394–395
4.	A	1	T2	Hales, p. 399
5.	C	1	T2	Hales, p. 401
6.	D	1	T3	Hales, p. 402
7.	B	1	T2	Hales, p. 402
8.	C	1	V1	Video
9.	B	1	V2	Video
10.	C	2	V3	Video
11.	nongonococcal urethritis	1	T1	Hales, p. 393
12.	condyloma	1	V2	Video
13.	F	1	V1	Video
14.	F	1	V2	Video
15.	T	2	V3	Video

Lesson 14

Cardiovascular Disease

I was lying there on the table and they were taking my blood pressure and in the course of doing that, something profoundly occurred and I began to slip away. It was clear to me . . . there was a lightness, an unexperienced lightness. I said to a person over me, "I'm gonna die. . . ."

—Charles Wolfe, describing his heart attack

LESSON ASSIGNMENT

Review the following assignment in order to schedule your time appropriately. Pay careful attention; the titles and numbers of the textbook chapter, the telecourse guide lesson, and the video program may be different from one another.

Text:

Hales, *An Invitation to Health,*
Chapter 12, "Keeping Your Heart Healthy," pp. 408–440. It will be helpful if you read the entire chapter before beginning this lesson.

Video:

"Cardiovascular Disease,"
from the series *Living with Health.*

OVERVIEW

If you read newspaper obituaries, often you will see the expression, "died suddenly," referring to people who die of heart attacks. If we really think about this, we realize that this usually is not an accurate description of what happened. Cardiovascular disease usually is not sudden at all. It develops slowly and insidiously for many years, and is only sudden when it manifests itself as a full-blown heart attack. The process has been developing for a long time, since our early years, we just did not know it. For this reason, knowledge about cardiovascular disease and its prevention is crucial to our health.

The two lessons relating to cardiovascular disease will cover the various dimensions of the problem. The development of the problems associated with cardiovascular diseases, the risk factors as well as the treatment and prevention of the various cardiovascular diseases will help us understand the group of diseases known to be the nation's top killer.

In order to understand the cardiovascular diseases, it is important to understand something about the anatomy and physiology of the heart and circulatory system. Remember the heart is a pump sending the blood to the various organs. The blood vessels form the pipelines that carry the blood. Arteries carry blood (usually oxygenated) away from the heart, and veins carry deoxygenated blood back to the heart. The exception to this is the pulmonary circulation. The pulmonary arteries carry deoxygenated blood to the lungs, where it is oxygenated before being returned to the heart via the pulmonary veins. Understanding this will help you see what can happen when the vessels become narrowed by disease, or when the heart is not pumping as effectively as it should.

Some of the most common and most important cardiovascular diseases are hypertension (high blood pressure), atherosclerosis, stroke, and myocardial infarction (heart attack). Yet, we can effectively lower our risk of these same diseases through lifestyle modification. The major risk factors for these diseases are smoking; obesity; a high fat, high salt diet; high blood cholesterol levels; cocaine use; lack of exercise; a family history of disease; and high blood pressure.

Because most of these cardiovascular conditions are relatively silent until they become quite far advanced, it is very important to pay attention if any of the danger signs appear. You should have your blood pressure checked on a regular basis. Any chest pain, shortness of breath, dizziness, indigestion, or heartburn should be evaluated by a physician. Too often we find that people deny the symptoms of cardiovascular disease until it is too late. If a person is having a heart attack, there is no time for delay. Time is critical to survival. Even if you "really don't" think this possibly could be a heart attack, it is essential to have it checked out.

LEARNING OBJECTIVES

Goal

You should be able to explain the cardiovascular diseases, the development of the diseases over time, and the risk factors associated with these diseases.

Objectives

Upon completion of this lesson, you should be able to:

1. Describe the anatomy and physiology of the heart and circulatory system, and explain hypertension and atherosclerosis as diseases and as causes of cardiovascular disease.

2. Discuss the following major cardiovascular conditions and diseases: elevated cholesterol, heart attack, stroke, transient ischemic attack, arrhythmias, congestive heart failure, rheumatic fever, and congenital defects. Describe the risk factors for each.

KEY TERMS

Look for these items as you proceed through the lesson assignments. Be able to discuss them upon completion of this lesson.

atrium
ventricles
systole
diastole
aorta
capillaries
arteriosclerosis
atherosclerosis
angina pectoris
myorcardial infarction (MI)
angioplasty
cardiopulmonary resuscitation (CPR)
tachycardia
bradycardia
atrial fibrillation
arrhythmia
congestive heart failure
stroke
transient ischemic attacks (TIAs)

TEXT FOCUS POINTS

The following focus points are designed to help you get the most from the text. Review them, then read the assignment. You may want to write notes to reinforce what you have learned.

Text: Hales, *An Invitation to Health*, Chapter 13, pp. 408–440.

1. Describe the anatomy of the heart and explain how blood flows through the heart and circulatory system.
2. Analyze the relationship of cholesterol to the risk of heart attack.
3. Define hypertension and list its common risk factors.
4. What are arteriosclerosis and atherosclerosis? How is atherosclerosis related to heart attack and how is it treated?
5. Explain what happens during a myocardial infarction (heart attack) and what can be done to treat and prevent such attacks.
6. List and explain some of the other major cardiovascular diseases.
7. Define stroke and transient ischemic attacks (TIAs) and explain their cause, treatment, and prevention.

VIDEO FOCUS POINTS

The following focus points are designed to help you get the most from the video segment of this lesson. Review them, then watch the video. You may want to write notes to reinforce what you have learned.

Video: "Cardiovascular Disease"

1. Explain the risk factors that increase one's chances of cardiovascular disease.
2. What changes in the cardiovascular system contribute to the actual heart attack?

INDIVIDUAL HEALTH PLAN

This portion of the lesson is designed to enable you to use the information you have learned in your own life situation to improve the quality of your life. You should do any exercise assigned, complete the journal portion of the plan, then put this portion of the health plan into practice in your life.

> Complete the Self-Survey, "Check Your Cholesterol and Heart Disease I.Q. on page 427 of your textbook. In your journal, list areas of your health, that you need to work on now that you understand the relationship of cholesterol to heart disease.

RELATED ACTIVITIES

These activities are not required unless your instructor assigns them. They are offered as suggestions to help you learn more about the material presented in this lesson.

1. Contact your college health center, local American Heart Association, or American Red Cross and take a cardiopulmonary resuscitation (CPR) class.

PRACTICE TEST

After reading the assignment and watching the video, you should be able to answer the Practice Test questions. Tests also include essay questions that are similar to the Textbook Focus Points and the Video Focus Points. When you have completed the Practice Test questions, turn to the Answer Key to score your answers.

Multiple-Choice

Select the one choice that best answers the question.

1. The term cardiovascular refers to __________.
   A. the heart and lungs
   B. the heart and blood vessels
   C. the heart and brain
   D. the brain and blood vessels

2. What is the largest major artery of the body?
   A. Pulmonary artery
   B. Femoral artery
   C. Aorta
   D. Superior vena cava

3. All of the following statements about cholesterol testing are true EXCEPT __________.
   A. test results are best measured after a fasting period
   B. getting more than one reading is always advisable before making decisions
   C. some medications may influence cholesterol readings
   D. samples are best drawn in a standing position from the finger

4. Hypertension has been identified as an increased risk for the development of all of the following diseases EXCEPT __________.
   A. vision problems
   B. osteoporosis
   C. heart disease
   D. kidney disease

5. All of the following lifestyle changes may influence the reversal of coronary artery disease EXCEPT __________.
   A. aerobic exercise
   B. relaxation techniques
   C. very low-fat diets
   D. drug therapies

6. Chest pain caused by a temporary inadequate supply of oxygen to the heart muscle is known as __________.
   A. angina pectoris
   B. myocardial infarction
   C. angioplasty
   D. hypertension

7. All of the following might be good strategies to employ in case you or someone you know might be experiencing a heart attack EXCEPT __________.
   A. training yourself in CPR
   B. waiting at least 15 minutes to be sure it's an actual heart attack
   C. knowing the EMS code in your area
   D. being prepared for symptoms of denial that it is a heart attack

8. The most common congenital defects that occur in the heart are __________.
   A. large ventricles
   B. transposed arteries
   C. missing valves
   D. holes in the ventricular septum

9. All of the following are true statements regarding the risk for development of stroke EXCEPT __________.
   A. men are at higher risk than women for stroke
   B. ethnicity may play a role in stroke risk
   C. an aspirin a day will diminish your risk of stroke
   D. heart attack and stroke are not related diseases

10. Factors that place the individual at higher risk for cardiovascular disease include all the following EXCEPT __________.
    A. smoking
    B. high salt diet
    C. sedentary lifestyle
    D. low-fat diet

11. Cardiovascular changes that lead to disease include all the following EXCEPT __________.
    A. narrowing vessels
    B. increasing blood pressure
    C. slowing heart rate
    D. developing plaque

Fill-in-the-Blank

Insert the correct word or words in the blank for each item.

12. The lower pumping chambers of the heart muscle are known as the ______________.

13. The medical name for a heart attack is ____________ ____________.

14. Lifestyle behaviors such as smoking and a high-fat diet, which increase one's chances for cardiovascular disease, are termed ________ __________.

15. When there is occlusion of the coronary arteries, the portion of the heart supplied by those arteries ________.

True-False

If the statement is true, write "T" to the left of the statement. If the statement (or any part of the statement) is false, write "F" to the left of the statement.

16. A diet low in salt and high in fat can decrease the risk for cardiovascular disease.

17. Hypertension is quite different from high blood pressure and presents may symptoms as soon as it occurs.

18. Cardiovascular changes leading to a heart attack occur very suddenly.

ANSWER KEY

The following provides the answers and references for the Practice Test questions. Focus Points are referenced using the following abbreviations:

T = Text and V = Video

	Answers	Learning Objectives	Focus Points	References
1.	B	1	T1	Hales, Pp. 410–414
2.	C	1	T1	Hales, p. 410
3.	D	1	T2	Hales, p. 419
4.	B	1	T3	Hales, p. 422
5.	D	1	T4	Hales, p. 426
6.	A	2	T5	Hales, p. 428
7.	B	2	T5	Hales, p. 430
8.	D	2	T6	Hales, p. 431
9.	D	2	T7	Hales, p. 436
10.	D	2	V1	Video
11.	C	2	V2	Video
12.	ventricles	1	T1	Hales, p. 410
13.	myocardial infarction	2	T5	Hales, p. 428
14.	risk factors	2	V1	Video
15.	dies	2	V2	Video
16.	F	2	V1	Video
17.	F	2	V2	Video
18.	F	2	V2	Video

Lesson 15

Treatment and Prevention of Cardiovascular Disease

Perhaps the question we should ask ourselves is not "Am I healthy?" but "Am I as healthy as I know how to be?" I believe that for almost all persons the answer would be an unequivocal "no." Almost everyone knows how to implement a higher order of healthiness. And if a "no" answer doesn't make us unmistakably uncomfortable, it is likely that we haven't squarely asked it. Answering "no" means we have hidden from ourselves. We have shunned an inner wisdom.

—Larry Dossey, M.D., *Beyond Illness*

LESSON ASSIGNMENT

Review the following assignment in order to schedule your time appropriately. Pay careful attention; the titles and numbers of the textbook chapter, the telecourse guide lesson, and the video program may be different from one another.

Text:

Hales, *An Invitation to Health,*
Chapter 12, "Keeping Your Heart Healthy," pp. 408–440. Review the chapter.

Video:

"Treatment and Prevention of Cardiovascular Disease"
from the series *Living with Health.*

OVERVIEW

While modern medicine has brought much hope for victims of cardiovascular disease, the most important treatment is actual prevention of the problem. Nowhere are our lifestyle decisions more important than in this group of diseases. While some of our risk factors are uncontrollable, most of those things that put us at higher risk for cardiovascular diseases can be controlled. Of even more concern is the way in which risk factors tend to multiply and reinforce each other. Somehow, if we have one bad lifestyle habit, we tend to have several which impact each other. If we are overweight, we tend not to exercise. If we smoke, we smoke even more when we are under stress. The good news is that good lifestyle habits tend to reinforce each other as well. When we exercise and eat in a healthy way, we lose weight and frequently handle stress more effectively.

The sooner we make decisions to improve our health, the sooner we lower our risks for cardiovascular and other diseases. Bad habits can be difficult to break, but if we do not become discouraged, we will reap the benefits of our work. We don't even have to do all things at once. We can work on our risks one by one. The important thing is that we begin. We will feel better, be healthier, and will have less risk of developing cardiovascular problems.

LEARNING OBJECTIVES

Goal

You should be able to identify and discuss methods of treatment of cardiovascular diseases and lifestyle behaviors that lower the risk of cardiovascular disease.

Objectives

Upon completion of this lesson, you should be able to:

1. Discuss the uncontrollable and controllable risk factors for cardiovascular disease, the danger of multiple risk factors, and ways the controllable risk factors can be reduced.

2. Identify and discuss the tests and treatments for cardiovascular disease which are used most frequently and the issues in recovery from cardiovascular disease.

KEY TERMS

Look for these items as you proceed through the lesson assignments. Be able to discuss them upon completion of this lesson.

antioxidants
hypertension
cholesterol
triglyceride
lipoproteins
male pattern baldness
electrocardiogram (ECG, EKG)
thallium scintigraphy
coronary angiography
coronary bypass
percutaneous transluminal coronary angioplasty (PTCA)

TEXT FOCUS POINTS

The following focus points are designed to help you get the most from the text. Review them, then read the assignment. You may want to write notes to reinforce what you have learned.

Text: Hales, *An Invitation to Health*, Chapter 12, pp. 408–440.

1. List and explain the controllable and uncontrollable risk factors for cardiovascular disease.
2. Discuss the most frequently used tests and treatments for cardiovascular disease.
3. What are the most important lifestyle behaviors one can do to lower the risk of cardiovascular disease?

VIDEO FOCUS POINTS

The following focus points are designed to help you get the most from the video segment of this lesson. Review them, then watch the video. You may want to write notes to reinforce what you have learned.

Video: "Treatment and Prevention of Cardiovascular Disease"

1. Why is having the knowledge of cardiopulmonary resuscitation (CPR) so important to the individual?
2. Discuss the various treatments for cardiovascular disease: medication, angioplasty, bypass surgery, and transplant.
3. What are some of the emotional and physical aspects involved in recovery from a heart attack?
4. What lifestyle choices and behaviors are important in lowering the individual's risk for cardiovascular disease? How are these important?

INDIVIDUAL HEALTH PLAN

This portion of the lesson is designed to enable you to use the information you have learned in your own life situation to improve the quality of your life. You should do any exercise assigned, complete the journal portion of the plan, then put this portion of the health plan into practice in your life.

> After assessing your risk factors for cardiovascular disease, develop a plan in your journal for lowering these risks using information you have gained in this lesson. Take action on your plan today.

RELATED ACTIVITIES

These activities are not required unless your instructor assigns them. They are offered as suggestions to help you learn more about the material presented in this lesson.

1. Design a cardiovascular risk reduction program for your own family based on your individual and family risks.

PRACTICE TEST

After reading the assignment and watching the video, you should be able to answer the Practice Test questions. Tests also include essay questions that are similar to the Text Focus Points and the Video Focus Points. When you have completed the Practice Test questions, turn to the Answer Key to score your answers.

Multiple-Choice

Select the one choice that best answers the question.

1. Which of the following activities would most likely be the best to engage in to decrease your risk of heart disease?
   A. Weight training
   B. Bowling
   C. Billiards
   D. Brisk walking

2. Which one of the following emotions has been most closely associated with an increased risk for heart disease?
   A. Depression
   B. Guilt
   C. Jealousy
   D. Anger

3. The testing procedure performed that involves the injection of radioactive isotopes into the bloodstream is known as __________.
   A. electrocardiogram
   B. thallium scintigraphy
   C. coronary angiography
   D. coronary angioplasty

4. Deaths from cardiovascular disease have decreased because of the following EXCEPT __________.
   A. a vegetarian diet.
   B. better surgical techniques.
   C. less smoking.
   D. more exercise.

5. Cardiopulmonary resuscitation (CPR) should be learned by __________.
   A. health care professionals
   B. food service workers
   C. everyone
   D. police and fire officers

6. When the heart is damaged beyond repair, the patient may have to consider __________.
   A. open heart repair
   B. heart transplant
   C. angioplasty
   D. bypass surgery

7. After a heart attack, the individual frequently has all the following EXCEPT __________.
   A. few emotional concerns
   B. changed dietary habits
   C. significant physical rehabilitation
   D. lifestyle adjustments

8. Hypertension is the same thing as __________.
   A. hyperactivity
   B. angioplasty
   C. atherosclerosis
   D. high blood pressure.

Fill-in-the-Blank

Insert the correct word or words in the blank for each item.

9. Foods that help prevent heart disease by protecting the heart from the harmful effects of cell damage are known as _______________.

10. The most accurate diagnostic testing procedure is a ___________ ___________.

11. When a balloon-type apparatus is threaded through the blood vessels to remove a blockage, the procedure is known as __________________.

12. The procedure in which the heart is removed and replaced by one from another person is called _______________.

True-False

If the statement is true, write "T" to the left of the statement. If the statement (or any part of the statement) is false, write "F" to the left of the statement.

13. CPR is important because it can maintain the supply of oxygen to the brain and vital organs.

14. Hypertension is usually treated with medication, a low-salt diet, and exercise.

15. The presence of multiple risk factors enormously increases one's risk of cardiovascular disease.

16. Exercise lowers the risk of cardiovascular disease by strengthening the skeletal system.

ANSWER KEY

The following provides the answers and references for the Practice Test questions. Focus Points are referenced using the following abbreviations:

T = Text and V = Video

	Answers	Learning Objectives	Focus Points	References
1.	D	1	T1	Hales, p. 411
2.	D	1	T1	Hales, p. 415
3.	B	2	T2	Hales, p. 432
4.	A	1	T3	Hales, pp. 432–434
5.	C	2	V1	Video
6.	B	2	V2	Video
7.	A	2	V3	Video
8.	D	1	V4	Video
9.	antioxidants	1	T1	Hales, p. 411
10.	coronary angiography	2	T2	Hales, p. 432
11.	angioplasty	2	V2	Video
12.	transplant	2	V2	Video
13.	T	2	V1	Video
14.	T	2	V2	Video
15.	T	1	V4	Video
16.	F	1	V4	Video

Lesson 16

Cancer

I'm living today with as much empowerment as I can and trying to help others. . . . I'm taking today a day at a time and I feel very good about that, so how much future does anybody have, mine's as good as yours.

—Beatrice Quintero, Cancer Survivor

LESSON ASSIGNMENT

Review the following assignment in order to schedule your time appropriately. Pay careful attention; the titles and numbers of the textbook chapter, the telecourse guide lesson, and the video program may be different from one another.

Text:

Hales, *An Invitation to Health*,
Chapter 13, "Lowering Your Risk of Cancer and Other Major Diseases,"
pp. 442–473.

Video:

"Cancer"
from the series *Living with Health.*

OVERVIEW

When people think of cancer, they frequently experience fear and think of cancer as a death sentence. This is just not true, though too many people are still dying of cancer. We need to understand that most cancers are treatable, and many are curable. Even more important to us, many cancers are preventable. Practicing a lifestyle that minimizes our risk factors for cancer can dramatically decrease our chance of dying of cancer. These lifestyle behaviors that put us at risk for cancer are similar to the ones that place us at risk for other health problems: tobacco, alcohol, poor dietary habits, the use of certain drugs, and exposure to certain carcinogenic substances.

Of equal importance to us is the knowledge of the seven warning signs of cancer and the key role that early detection plays in the treatment of cancer. One of the real tragedies of cancer is that people often delay getting treatment. There are several reasons for this delay: fear, not recognizing the early warning signs, not practicing self-examination, etc. But whatever the reason, delay in detection and treatment decreases our chances for successful treatment and survival of cancer. If we are to maximize our chances of preventing cancer, as well as surviving it should we get it, we must first practice a healthy lifestyle that lowers our risk for the disease. We must know the seven warning signs and practice self-examination. Then if we experience symptoms that indicate any possibility of cancer, we must seek diagnosis and treatment from a qualified physician immediately! If we do these things we dramatically increase our chance for a healthy, cancer-free life!

Though cancer is probably the most feared of the major noninfectious diseases, people live each day with serious chronic diseases. Some cannot be prevented and are a factor of genetics and chance. Others are preventable, or at least partially so, with attention to lifestyle. This lesson helps us understand the causes, risk factors, development, diagnosis, and treatment of some of the most common noninfectious diseases. We will also learn more of the special needs of people with differences in physical and mental abilities.

LEARNING OBJECTIVES

Goal

You should be able to describe cancer, its development, classifications of tumors, risk factors, prevention, and treatment, and explain other major noninfective diseases and their treatment.

Objectives

Upon completion of this lesson, you should be able to:

1. Define cancer, its classification and development, the emotional and social effects, risk factors and ways to reduce those risks, and treatment of various types of cancer.

2. List the other major noninfective diseases, their symptoms, risk factors, and treatment.

KEY TERMS

Look for these items as you proceed through the lesson assignments. Be able to discuss them upon completion of this lesson.

neoplasm
infiltration
metastasize
oncogene
tumor suppressor genes
relative risk
carcinogen
chemoprevention
mammography
lumpectomy
quadrantectomy
mastectomy
tamoxifen
bone marrow transplantation
gene therapy
diabetes mellitus
epilepsy
asthma
chronic obstructive lung disease (COLD)
anemia
cirrhosis
nephrosis
kidney stones
ulcer
inflammatory bowel disease (IBD)
irritable bowel syndrome
gallstone
arthritis
hernia
dermatitis
psoriasis
rehabilitation medicine

TEXT FOCUS POINTS

The following focus points are designed to help you get the most from the text. Review them, then read the assignment. You may want to write notes to reinforce what you have learned.

Text: Hales, *An Invitation to Health*, Chapter 13, pp. 442–473.

1. Define cancer, explain its development, and discuss the various classifications of it.

2. List the seven warning signs of cancer and explain the risk factors for cancer. What are some of the practical ways to reduce the risks?

3. Describe the different forms of cancer and the appropriate treatments for each.

4. Define diabetes mellitus and describe the early symptoms and treatment for this disease.

5. List and explain other major noninfectious illnesses.

VIDEO FOCUS POINTS

The following focus points are designed to help you get the most from the video segment of this lesson. Review them, then watch the video. You may want to write notes to reinforce what you have learned.

Video: "Cancer"

1. Explain what cancer is, the major types of cancer, and how cancer spreads.

2. Explain the circumstances under which the three most common types of cancer treatment are used.

3. Describe three kinds of emotional issues cancer patients and their families must face relative to each patient's attitude toward treatment.

4. Discuss eight lifestyle behaviors that will decrease the individual's risk of cancer.

INDIVIDUAL HEALTH PLAN

This portion of the lesson is designed to enable you to use the information you have learned in your own life situation to improve the quality of your life. You should do any exercise assigned, complete the journal portion of the plan, then put this portion of the health plan into practice in your life.

> Complete the Self-Survey, "Are You at Risk of Cancer?" on page 451 in your textbook. In your journal, analyze what you have learned about your risks of cancer. Using what you have learned, analyze your risks for the other major noninfectious diseases. What can you do to decrease your risk for these diseases?

RELATED ACTIVITIES

These activities are not required unless your instructor assigns them. They are offered as suggestions to help you learn more about the material presented in this lesson.

1. Visit the local chapter of the American Cancer Society to find out what educational material and community services it provides. Consider volunteering in a program.

PRACTICE TEST

After reading the assignment and watching the video, you should be able to answer the Practice Test questions. Tests also include essay questions that are similar to the Text Focus Points and the Video Focus Points. When you have completed the Practice Test questions, turn to the Answer Key to score your answers.

Multiple-Choice

Select the one choice that best answers the question.

1. When cancer cells spread from their original site to other parts of the body via the bloodstream or lymph system, this is known as __________.
   A. metastasis
   B. infiltration
   C. malignancy
   D. invasion

2. All of the following are true statements regarding cancer and heredity EXCEPT __________.
   A. hereditary cancer usually strikes people at a younger age
   B. if your parent develops cancer, your risk for cancer is automatically greater
   C. similar types of cancer may attack family members at different sites
   D. rarer forms of cancer are not usually hereditary in nature

3. The surgery typically used to treat breast cancer where the whole of the breast tissue is removed is known as a __________.
   A. lumpectomy
   B. mastectomy
   C. quandrantectomy
   D. mammography

4. All of the following are true statements regarding diabetes EXCEPT ________.
   A. wounds heal very slowly in diabetics
   B. it always requires the administration of insulin
   C. it involves a condition of excessive glucose in bloodstream
   D. it may result in complications that lead to blindness

5. The primary cause of chronic obstructive lung diseases in the United States is __________.
   A. air pollution
   B. cigarette smoking
   C. asbestos exposure
   D. allergies

6. All of the following actions will likely increase your risk of developing back problems EXCEPT __________.
   A. having very poor posture while sitting at your desk
   B. not warming up before engaging in a strength workout
   C. sleeping at night on a firm, flat mattress
   D. being obese

7. Which of the following phrases does NOT describe cancer?
   A. Group of diseases
   B. Generally untreatable
   C. Capable of metastatic growth
   D. Problem of regulation and differentiation of cells

8. Most cancers are treated using __________.
   A. surgery
   B. radiation
   C. chemotherapy
   D. combinations of treatments

9. Which of the following lifestyle behaviors will NOT decrease the risk of cancer?
   A. Not smoking
   B. Abstaining from alcohol
   C. Getting a good suntan
   D. Eating a high fiber diet

Fill-in-the-Blank

Insert the correct word or words in the blank for each item.

10. Cancers which originate in epithelial tissue are known as ____________.

11. The disease that occurs when the body cannot produce or effectively use insulin is known as ____________ ____________.

12. More than 17 million people have some form of __________, an inflammatory disease of the joints that takes over a hundred forms.

13. Cancers that arise in the blood-forming tissues are leukemias and ____________________.

14. A test which contributes to lowering the risk of dying from breast cancer is the ____________________.

True-False

If the statement is true, write "T" to the left of the statement. If the statement (or any part of the statement) is false, write "F" to the left of the statement.

15. Localized tumors are usually treated with chemotherapy.

16. When the diagnosis of cancer is made, most people respond with shock, denial, or even anger.

ANSWER KEY

The following provides the answers and references for the Practice Test questions. Focus Points are referenced using the following abbreviations:
T = Text and V = Video

	Answers	Learning Objectives	Focus Points	References
1.	A	1	T1	Hales, p. 444
2.	D	1	T2	Hales, p. 445
3.	B	1	T3	Hales, p. 457
4.	B	2	T4	Hales, p. 463
5.	B	2	T5	Hales, p. 465
6.	C	2	T5	Hales, p. 469
7.	B	1	V1	Video
8.	D	1	V2	Video
9.	C	1	V4	Video
10.	carcinomas	1	T1	Hales, p. 444
11.	diabetes mellitus	2	T4	Hales, p. 462
12.	arthritis	2	T5	Hales, p. 468
13.	lymphomas	1	V1	Video
14.	mammogram	1	V4	Video
15.	F	1	V2	Video
16.	T	1	V3	Video

Lesson 17

Drugs

The mental and spiritual qualities of man will never be dignified through debasing the physical and vice versa. This understanding is crucial to the maturation of a holistic theory of health. . . .

—Larry Dossey, M.D., *Beyond Illness*

LESSON ASSIGNMENT

Review the following assignment in order to schedule your time appropriately. Pay careful attention; the titles and numbers of the textbook chapter, the telecourse guide lesson, and the video program may be different from one another.

Text:

Hales, *An Invitation to Health,*
Chapter 14, "Drug Use, Misuse, and Abuse," pp. 476–511.
Review Chapter 4, "The Joy of Fitness," pp. 126–128.

Video:

"Drugs"
from the series *Living with Health.*

OVERVIEW

At the same time that we are so concerned with drug abuse, we must look at the environment in which this abuse is taking place. We have to face the fact that we are a drug-oriented society. All we have to do is turn on our television or open a magazine to realize that "there is a pill for everything." While many drugs save lives and are absolutely necessary to our health and well-being, some of these and many others are overused, misused, abused, and present major health problems.

Many of the reasons that cause people to misuse and abuse drugs, including alcohol, relate to two concepts. One is the relief of pain, whether it be physical, emotional, or social. The other is an attempt to make life different, to be accepted, to fit in, to be happy, etc. If we consider this, we will see that there are always more positive means to achieve these objectives. This is what making healthy lifestyle decisions is all about. Coping with the ups and downs of life certainly is not always easy, but while drug use may seem a simple solution for the present, it creates havoc in the longer term. The negative health effects on the individual, his or her family, and even future generations is just not worth the momentary high.

Drug misuse and abuse crosses all socioeconomic, ethnic, gender, and age lines. There is not a typical drug abuser. No one is "immune" to the risk. If you or someone you care about is having a problem, get help. Now is the time for each of us to take the responsibility for making decisions for health. In addition to preventing or solving problems for ourselves, we can help solve a greater community problem, because as the demand for drugs decreases, so does the illegal drug trade and its societal problems.

LEARNING OBJECTIVES

Goal

You should be able to discuss the various factors influencing drug use, misuse, and abuse; the substance use disorders; common drugs of abuse; and treatment of drug dependency.

Objectives

Upon completion of this lesson, you should be able to:

1. Explain the factors influencing drug use, misuse, and dependency, and the scope of drug-related problems in the United States.

2. Describe the common drugs of abuse; their use, effects, and risks; and the treatment of drug dependency and abuse.

KEY TERMS

Look for these items as you proceed through the lesson assignments. Be able to discuss them upon completion of this lesson.

drug
drug misuse
drug abuse
inhalants
intravenous
intramuscular
subcutaneous
set
toxicity
additive
synergistic
potentiating
antagonistic
over-the-counter (OTC) drugs
noncompliance
generic
psychotropic
stimulant
psychoactive
addiction
psychological dependence
physical dependence
intoxication
withdrawal
polyabuse
amphetamines
hashish
marijuana
cocaine
hallucinogen
deleriants
opioids
nonopioids
PCP (phencyclidine)
benzodiazepines
barbiturates
anabolic steroids
GHB/gamma hydroxybutyrate
GBL/gamma butyrolactone
designer drugs
twelve-step program
codependence

TEXT FOCUS POINTS

The following focus points are designed to help you get the most from the text. Review them, then read the assignment. You may want to write notes to reinforce what you have learned.

Text: Hales, *An Invitation to Health*, Chapter 14, pp. 476–511. Review Chapter 4, pp. 126–128.

1. Explain the factors affecting drug use and misuse.
2. Distinguish among the substance use disorders. What are some of the causes of drug dependence and abuse?
3. Discuss the scope of the problems of drug use in the United States today.
4. Describe the common drugs of abuse including amphetamines, cocaine, hallucinogens, inhalants, opioids, PCP, sedative-hypnotic drugs, anabolic steroids, and the designer drugs. Include the methods of use, effects, and risks associated with each.
5. Describe the methods of treating drug dependence and abuse and the factors affecting treatment, including codependence.

VIDEO FOCUS POINTS

The following focus points are designed to help you get the most from the video segment of this lesson. Review them, then watch the video. You may want to write notes to reinforce what you have learned.

Video: "Drugs"

1. Describe the risks of and alternatives to anabolic steroid use.
2. Discuss the problems of drug abuse in society today. What are some of the decisions that have to be made if the problems of drug abuse are to be solved?
3. What are the risks and problems associated with the interaction of alcohol with other drugs and combinations of drugs?

INDIVIDUAL HEALTH PLAN

This portion of the lesson is designed to enable you to use the information you have learned in your own life situation to improve the quality of your life. You should do any exercise assigned, complete the journal portion of the plan, then put this portion of the health plan into practice in your life.

> Complete the Self-Survey, "Is It a Substance Use Disorder?" on page 486 of your textbook. Was there anything about this that surprised you? In your journal, examine the role that drugs play in your life. Consider the positive uses (antibiotics, etc.) as well as possible negatives. Include caffeine and any other "everyday" substance that you might not think of as a drug. Are there changes you should make to be healthier? What decisions will you need to make? What are some positive alternatives? If you feel that you are having a problem, consult your physician, your college health center, or your local Council on Alcoholism and Drug Abuse.

RELATED ACTIVITIES

These activities are not required unless your instructor assigns them. They are offered as suggestions to help you learn more about the material presented in this lesson.

1. Visit several drug treatment centers in your city and find out about their programs. Compare and contrast their approaches, cost, etc.

PRACTICE TEST

After reading the assignment and watching the video, you should be able to answer the Practice Test questions. Tests also include essay questions that are similar to the Text Focus Points and the Video Focus Points. When you have completed the Practice Test questions, turn to the Answer Key to score your answers.

Multiple-Choice

Select the one choice that best answers the question.

1. Injecting drugs beneath the skin is an example of __________.
   A. intravenous injection
   B. intramuscular injection
   C. subcutaneous injection
   D. huffing

2. A drug that continues to build up in the body, because it is accumulating faster than it can be metabolized, such as alcohol, is acting __________.
   A. locally
   B. selectively
   C. generally
   D. cumulatively

3. The term psychotropic means __________.
   A. illegal for use and purchase
   B. mind-affecting
   C. psychologically addicting
   D. causes psychotic behavior

4. All of the following are probably true statements regarding drug prevention in the United States EXCEPT __________.
   A. programs that emphasize resistance to peer pressure do work
   B. a supportive community around the addict increases likelihood of success
   C. education will only work with a corresponding change in drug attitudes
   D. stopping addiction is easier if more burden is placed on the addict

5. Propylexedrine or crank is commonly found in __________.
   A. diet pills
   B. decongestant inhalers
   C. antianxiety drugs
   D. marijuana

6. Opioid-based drugs are commonly prescribed as __________.
   A. antitoxins
   B. pain killers
   C. anxiety reducers
   D. all of the above are correct

7. What is probably the most difficult step for the individual to take to achieve successful recovery from addiction?
   A. Getting through physical withdrawal effects
   B. Becoming accustomed to and avoiding cravings
   C. Admitting to being an addict
   D. Overcoming the psychological problems that all those with addictive behaviors possess

8. Risks of anabolic steroids do NOT include __________.
   A. cancer of the liver
   B. heart problems
   C. personality disorders
   D. tuberculosis

9. Categories for describing usage of drugs would NOT include __________.
   A. biological
   B. medical
   C. social/psychological
   D. political

10. The interaction of sedative/tranquilizer drugs and alcohol causes __________.
   A. each drug to be less effective
   B. significant potentiation/synergistic effects
   C. very predictable effects
   D. no problem that either drug would not cause by itself

Fill-in-the-Blank

Insert the correct word or words in the blank for each item.

11. The dosage level at which most drugs become poisonous is referred to as the ___________ level.

12. The need for a larger and larger dose to achieve the same effect with a drug defines ___________.

13. ___________ ___________ are drugs that are synthetic derivatives of the male sex hormone testosterone.

14. The genetic predisposition of an individual to abuse drugs is a ______________ __________.

True-False

If the statement is true, write "T" to the left of the statement. If the statement (or any part of the statement) is false, write "F" to the left of the statement.

15. Most anabolic steroid use occurs among college and professional athletes.

16. The incidence of drug abuse is lower among individuals who come from dysfunctional families.

17. Most times, the effects of the interaction of alcohol and other depressant drugs is just slightly greater than the effect of either drug alone.

ANSWER KEY

The following provides the answers and references for the Practice Test questions. Focus Points are referenced using the following abbreviations:

T = Text and V = Video

	Answers	Learning Objectives	Focus Points	References
1.	C	1	T1	Hales, p. 478
2.	D	1	T1	Hales, p. 479
3.	B	1	T2	Hales, p. 483
4.	D	1	T3	Hales, pp. 488 and pp. 507–508
5.	B	2	T4	Hales, p. 492
6.	B	2	T4	Hales, p. 501
7.	C	2	T5	Hales, p. 505
8.	D	2	V1	Video
9.	D	2	V2	Video
10.	B	2	V3	Video
11.	toxicity	1	T1	Hales, p. 478
12.	tolerance	1	T2	Hales, p. 486
13.	Anabolic steroids	2	T4	Hales, p. 126
14.	biological factor	2	V2	Video
15.	F	2	V1	Video
16.	F	2	V2	Video
17.	F	2	V3	Video

Lesson 18

Alcohol

In American society, one of the biggest factors that contributes to people drinking is that alcohol is not seen as a drug. It's in some ways seen as a rite of passage.

—Robin LaDue, Ph.D.

LESSON ASSIGNMENT

Review the following assignment in order to schedule your time appropriately. Pay careful attention; the titles and numbers of the textbook chapter, the telecourse guide lesson, and the video program may be different from one another.

Text:

Hales, *An Invitation to Health*,
Chapter 15 "Alcohol Use, Misuse, and Abuse," pp. 512–541.

Video:

"Alcohol"
from the series *Living with Health.*

OVERVIEW

Alcohol has a strange history. Nearly 50 percent or half of all adults in the United States drink and 90 percent of college students use alcohol. On one hand it is accepted and even expected at many celebrations; on the other, it is the most abused of all drugs and causes enormous health problems. The obvious question is, "Why?" Why do some people use alcohol all their lives without experiencing any difficulties while others develop problems of great magnitude? The answers are varied and complex. What we do know is that excessive use of alcohol, even minimal amounts (as in the case of the pregnant woman) can cause significant damage to most body systems. Alcohol also plays an important role in violence of all kinds, from motor vehicle accidents to murder.

To make decisions about our own lifestyle in relationship to alcohol, it is important for us to understand the effects of alcohol on the body. Alcohol acts as an anesthetic, a sedative, and a depressant. This means that even small amounts are risky if we are doing anything that requires us to be alert. Small amounts of alcohol can also damage the developing fetus, so pregnant women are encouraged to abstain from alcohol use. A decision not to use alcohol certainly lowers our risk for problems, but it is also possible to use alcohol responsibly if we choose to. The important thing is that if we use alcohol, we use it responsibly so as not to cause harm to ourselves or others.

It has been said that you have an alcohol problem if your use of alcohol causes problems to you, your loved ones, your job, or any aspect of your life. This is a good measure if you think you or someone you care about seems to be developing alcohol problems. If you suspect alcohol problems may exist, there are many places to get help. Alcoholics Anonymous is the best known, but most cities have a variety of options for seeking help.

If you understand the effects and potential risks of alcohol use, you can make wise lifestyle decisions, whether you choose to abstain from alcohol or use alcohol in a responsible way.

LEARNING OBJECTIVES

Goal

You should be able to explain the significance of alcohol use in this country, the factors that influence alcohol use, the health and behavior consequences of alcohol abuse, alcohol treatment, and the responsible use of alcohol.

Objectives

Upon completion of this lesson, you should be able to:

1. Describe the effects of alcohol on the body, the factors that affect the response to alcohol, and the patterns of alcohol use and misuse in the United States.

2. Discuss alcoholism, its symptoms, causes, treatment programs, and negative impacts on family members and others.

KEY TERMS

Look for these items as you proceed through the lesson assignments. Be able to discuss them upon completion of this lesson.

ethyl alcohol
proof
blood-alcohol concentration (BAC)
absorption
intoxication
fetal alcohol syndrome (FAS)
fetal alcohol effects (FAE)
alcohol abuse
alcohol dependence
alcoholism
detoxification
delirium tremens (DTs)
relapse prevention
codependence

TEXT FOCUS POINTS

The following focus points are designed to help you get the most from the text. Review them, then read the assignment. You may want to write notes to reinforce what you have learned.

Text: Hales, *An Invitation to Health*, Chapter 15, pp. 512–541.

1. Describe the factors affecting a drinker's response to alcohol consumption.

2. How does alcohol affect the different body systems? How can it interact with other drugs?

3. Describe the patterns of alcohol use occurring in the United States today. What impact does alcohol misuse have on students, women, and different ethnic groups?

4. Define alcoholism and list common symptoms of this disease. Include some of the causes, types, and medical complications.

5. Explain the common methods of treatment for alcohol problems.

6. What are some of the negative impacts of alcohol abuse on family members and others in society?

VIDEO FOCUS POINTS

The following focus points are designed to help you get the most from the video segment of this lesson. Review them, then watch the video. You may want to write notes to reinforce what you have learned.

Video: "Alcohol"

1. Describe how social and psychological factors influence alcohol use and can place the individual consuming alcohol at risk.
2. Describe the progression toward alcoholism and some of the signs of alcoholism.
3. How is alcohol related to accidents and other violence?
4. What are some important considerations in the responsible use of alcohol?

INDIVIDUAL HEALTH PLAN

This portion of the lesson is designed to enable you to use the information you have learned in your own life situation to improve the quality of your life. You should do any exercise assigned, complete the journal portion of the plan, then put this portion of the health plan into practice in your life.

> Compare your own alcohol use with the levels in the Self-Survey, "Do You Have a Drinking Problem?" on page 532 of your textbook. Record your findings in your journal. Are there things that surprise you? Concern you? What did you learn about your patterns of alcohol use? If you found that there are times that you use alcohol irresponsibly, what will it take to change this pattern? Consider making some responsible decisions. If you discovered things that concerned you, discuss these with your college counseling or health center staff, your physician, or some other health professional.
>
> Note: If you do not use alcohol, discuss the reasons that led you to make the decision to abstain from alcohol use.

RELATED ACTIVITIES

These activities are not required unless your instructor assigns them. They are offered as suggestions to help you learn more about the material presented in this lesson.

1. Visit an open AA meeting and find out how the concept of a twelve-step program works.

2. Contact several alcohol treatment programs and find out how they treat alcohol abuse.

3. Interview a recovering alcoholic and find out how life has progressed before, during, and since alcohol abuse.

PRACTICE TEST

After reading the assignment and watching the video, you should be able to answer the Practice Test questions. Tests also include essay questions that are similar to the Text Focus Points and the Video Focus Points. When you have completed the Practice Test questions, turn to the Answer Key to score your answers.

Multiple-Choice

Select the one choice that best answers the question.

1. The most widely used mind-altering substance in the world is __________.
   A. alcohol
   B. cocaine
   C. nicotine
   D. marijuana

2. Liver metabolization of alcohol takes place at a rate dependent upon _________.
   A. body size
   B. age and tolerance
   C. many variables
   D. no variables; it is a constant rate

3. All of the following are potential signs of alcohol intoxication in an individual EXCEPT _________.
   A. aggressive sexual behavior
   B. mood swings
   C. slurred speech
   D. heightened sense of awareness

4. All of the following are reported reasons why people choose to drink alcohol EXCEPT _________.
   A. to participate in celebrations
   B. to emulate their role models who drink
   C. to obtain a heightened sense of awareness
   D. to be at social ease around others

5. Which of the following vitamins has been identified as being dangerously deficient among alcoholics?
   A. Vitamin A
   B. Thiamine
   C. Niacin
   D. Vitamin C

6. Programs which provide a controlled environment for alcoholics during detoxification are _________.
   A. self-help groups
   B. outpatient treatments
   C. inpatient treatments
   D. family therapy programs

7. Reasons that people begin drinking do NOT include _________.
   A. peer pressure
   B. rite of passage
   C. taste of alcohol
   D. advertising

8. A major sign that alcohol is becoming a problem is __________.
   A. functioning effectively at work
   B. drinking on the weekend
   C. consuming hard liquor
   D. family members' recognition that there is a problem

Fill-in-the-Blank

Insert the correct word or words in the blank for each item.

9. Passage of alcohol into the body tissues is a variable rate based on factors that affect ______________.

10. The physical and mental defects caused by the ingestion of alcohol by a woman during pregnancy are referred to as __________ ___________ ____________.

11. Gradual withdrawal from alcohol, or _________________, is usually the first phase of treatment for alcohol dependence.

12. By enabling the addict in his/her dependence, and by being codependents, the family and friends of an alcoholic serve to reinforce the __________ of the addict that there is an alcohol problem.

13. The various stages of progression to alcoholism are called the alcoholic ________________.

True-False

If the statement is true, write "T" to the left of the statement. If the statement (or any part of the statement) is false, write "F" to the left of the statement.

14. People rarely begin to drink before young adulthood.

15. The tendency to progress toward alcoholism is limited to a narrow segment of the population.

16. Alcohol is involved in many motor vehicle accidents, but plays a lesser role in other violence.

17. Responsible use of alcohol can mean that the person abstains from alcohol completely.

ANSWER KEY

The following provides the answers and references for the Practice Test questions. Focus Points are referenced using the following abbreviations:

T = Text and V = Video

	Answers	Learning Objectives	Focus Points	References
1.	A	1	T1	Hales, p. 512
2.	D	1	T2	Hales, p. 517
3.	D	1	T1	Hales, p. 516
4.	C	1	T3	Hales, p. 520
5.	B	2	T4	Hales, p. 534
6.	C	2	T5	Hales, p. 535
7.	C	1	V1	Video
8.	D	2	V2	Video
9.	absorption	1	T1	Hales, p. 515
10.	fetal alcohol syndrome	1	T3	Hales, p. 529
11.	detoxification	2	T5	Hales, p. 535
12.	denial	2	T6	Hales, p. 537
13.	continuum	2	V2	Video
14.	F	1	V1	Video
15.	F	2	V2	Video
16.	F	1	V3	Video
17.	T	1	V4	Video

Lesson 19

Tobacco

If you can't breathe, nothing else matters.
—American Lung Association

LESSON ASSIGNMENT

Review the following assignment in order to schedule your time appropriately. Pay careful attention; the titles and numbers of the textbook chapter, the telecourse guide lesson, and the video program may be different from one another.

Text:

Hales, *An Invitation to Health*,
Chapter 16, "Tobacco Use, Misuse, and Abuse," pp. 542–565.

Video:

"Tobacco"
from the series *Living with Health.*

OVERVIEW

Tobacco use causes the most preventable illness and death in the United States today. Though tobacco advertisements still portray smoking as glamorous or macho, there is nothing glamorous or macho about the damage that tobacco does to the body. Death from the tobacco-related lung diseases is long and agonizing, with the patient gasping for each breath. The advertisements don't mention that, or the other problems associated with tobacco. Of particular concern is the effect of tobacco on children. From the problems caused in the unborn child to the increase in respiratory diseases experienced by the children of smoking parents, the effects of tobacco affect the innocent. The increased use of tobacco products by teens is also cause for grave concern.

The factors that cause people to start smoking and continue to smoke are varied, but of interest is the fact that most smokers would rather be nonsmokers. The addiction properties of nicotine are very strong indeed. This physical need added to the psychological one makes it very difficult to stop smoking. The risk of environmental tobacco smoke to the nonsmoker has been and is an important health issue. Efforts by the American Lung Association and other groups concerned with the effects of environmental tobacco smoke have also caused legislation prohibiting smoking in many areas, an important step in lowering the risk to nonsmokers.

Though we did not reach the goal of a smoke-free society by the year 2000, there are signs of hope that at some point in the future we will be able to study tobacco from a historical perspective rather than having to contend with it as a major health threat. In the meantime, if we can persuade our young people not to begin to smoke, we will be much closer to a truly healthy society.

LEARNING OBJECTIVES

Goal

You should be able to discuss the significance of tobacco use, the health consequences of tobacco use for the smoker and nonsmoker, ways to stop smoking, and ways in which the problems associated with tobacco use are being combatted.

Objectives

Upon completion of this lesson, you should be able to:

1. Explain the health effects of tobacco use, its relationship to various diseases, and the dangers of passive tobacco smoke.

2. Analyze the scope of tobacco use in the United States, the politics of tobacco, and ways to stop smoking and minimize its effects.

KEY TERMS

Look for these items as you proceed through the lesson assignments. Be able to discuss them upon completion of this lesson.

nicotine
tar
carbon monoxide
environmental tobacco smoke
bidis
mainstream smoke
sidestream smoke
aversion therapy
bupropion

TEXT FOCUS POINTS

The following focus points are designed to help you get the most from the text. Review them, then read the assignment. You may want to write notes to reinforce what you have learned.

Text: Hales, *An Invitation to Health*, Chapter 16, pp. 542–565.

1. List and describe the effects of tobacco on the body. What are the diseases and health effects related to tobacco use?

2. Describe today's typical tobacco smoker and the reasons that people begin to smoke and keep smoking.

3. Discuss the health effects of clove cigarettes, pipes, cigars, and smokeless tobacco.

4. What are the dangers of passive or environmental tobacco smoke?

5. Analyze the politics of tobacco. Include a strategy for keeping your personal environment smoke-free.

6. Describe several recommended ways to quit smoking.

VIDEO FOCUS POINTS

The following focus points are designed to help you get the most from the video segment of this lesson. Review them, then watch the video. You may want to write notes to reinforce what you have learned.

Video: "Tobacco"

1. Explain some of the social, psychological, and physiological factors that influence tobacco use.
2. Describe the effects of smoking on the nonsmoker, including the unborn child and children of smokers.
3. How does the tobacco industry attempt to replace smokers, particularly with women, minorities, and teenagers?
4. Describe some of the benefits of giving up smoking and the importance of not beginning to smoke.

INDIVIDUAL HEALTH PLAN

This portion of the lesson is designed to enable you to use the information you have learned in your own life situation to improve the quality of your life. You should do any exercise assigned, complete the journal portion of the plan, then put this portion of the health plan into practice in your life.

> If you are a smoker, complete the Self-Survey, "Are You Addicted to Nicotine?" on page 550 of your textbook. Using the information you have gained, write a stop-smoking plan for yourself in your journal. Now, carry out your plan. If you need additional help, contact the American Lung Association or American Cancer Society in your area.
>
> If you are a nonsmoker, list in your journal the times in your day that you are exposed to passive smoking. Plan ways in which you could reduce this exposure. Take action on your plan.

RELATED ACTIVITIES

These activities are not required unless your instructor assigns them. They are offered as suggestions to help you learn more about the material presented in this lesson.

1. If you have a friend or loved one who smokes, interview them and find out why they smoke, why it is hard for them to quit, and how they have tried to quit. See if there are ways that you might help them become nonsmokers if they want to.
2. Contact the American Lung Association, American Cancer Society, and/or the American Heart Association in your area and find out more about their programs related to tobacco use.
3. Find out about the Clean Indoor Air legislation that exists in your community. If none exists or if you don't think it is adequate, get involved with some of the groups trying to improve the quality of indoor air.

PRACTICE TEST

After reading the assignment and watching the video, you should be able to answer the Practice Test questions. Tests also include essay questions that are similar to the Text Focus Points and the Video Focus Points. When you have completed the Practice Test questions, turn to the Answer Key to score your answers.

Multiple-Choice

Select the one choice that best answers the question.

1. All of the following are physiological effects from nicotine use EXCEPT __________.
   A. constricts the blood vessels
   B. increases the need to urinate
   C. dulls the taste buds
   D. increases the heart rate

2. The leading cause of death from smoking-related causes annually is ________.
   A. heart disease
   B. lung cancer
   C. emphysema
   D. stroke

3. All of the following might be factors influencing people to start smoking EXCEPT __________.
   A. the influence of parental role models
   B. an aspect of adolescent rebellion
   C. a secondary factor to some other drug dependency
   D. aggressive marketing strategies by tobacco companies

4. The natural anesthetic in clove cigarettes that creates a long-term hazard for clove smokers is __________.
   A. Demerol
   B. eugenol
   C. Atavan
   D. estrogen

5. Exposure to the smoke that is coming off the end of a burning cigarette is __________.
   A. mainstream smoke
   B. sidestream smoke
   C. both mainstream and sidestream smoke
   D. none of the above

6. In the United States, airlines now prohibit smoking on all __________.
   A. flights under one hour long
   B. domestic flights
   C. flights, either foreign or domestic
   D. none of the above; there are no regulations in the airline industry

7. Quitting completely all at once is recommended to individuals who are ______.
   A. under age 30
   B. diabetic or have some other health concern
   C. heavily addicted
   D. overweight or obese

8. One of the reasons that people continue to smoke is that nicotine is _________.
   A. addicting
   B. pleasurable
   C. relatively harmless
   D. carcinogenic

9. Tobacco use by the pregnant woman can __________.
   A. produce little damage in the fetus
   B. result in a more difficult labor
   C. seriously affect the fetus
   D. cause liver failure in the fetus

10. The tobacco industry attempts to appeal to women and minorities by portraying smoking as all the following EXCEPT as __________.
    A. reality
    B. sophisticated
    C. healthy
    D. sexy

11. One of the main functions of smoking cessation group programs is that members receive __________.
    A. guaranteed results
    B. support from each other
    C. in-depth psychotherapy
    D. medication

Fill-in-the-Blank

Insert the correct word or words in the blank for each item.

12. The dark, sticky substance produced from the burning of tobacco is known as _______.

13. Finely ground tobacco that is placed inside the cheek and sucked is called __________.

14. The gum sometimes used by people attempting to quit smoking is known as __________ gum.

15. When a person is physically dependent on a drug like tobacco, the condition is termed ______________.

True-False

If the statement is true, write "T" to the left of the statement. If the statement (or any part of the statement) is false, write "F" to the left of the statement.

16. Babies born of mothers who smoke are frequently low in birth weight and experience other health problems.

17. The nicotine patch guarantees that the smoker will be able to stop smoking.

ANSWER KEY

The following provides the answers and references for the Practice Test questions. Focus Points are referenced using the following abbreviations:

T = Text and V = Video

	Answers	Learning Objectives	Focus Points	References
1.	B	1	T1	Hales, p. 544
2.	A	1	T1	Hales, p. 545
3.	C	2	T2	Hales, pp. 547–548
4.	B	1	T3	Hales, p. 555
5.	B	1	T4	Hales, p. 557
6.	B	2	T5	Hales, p. 558
7.	C	2	T6	Hales, p. 560
8.	A	1	V1	Video
9.	C	1	V2	Video
10.	A	2	V3	Video
11.	B	2	V4	Video
12.	tar	1	T1	Hales, p. 544
13.	snuff	1	T3	Hales, p. 556
14.	Nicorette	2	T6	Hales, p. 561
15.	addiction	1	V1	Video
16.	T	1	V2	Video
17.	F	2	V4	Video

Lesson 20

Injury Prevention

I can tell you from my perspective as a physician, seeing the tragedies of young people coming into our trauma centers with their severe injuries, multiple fractures, brain injury. . . I look upon the fact that these are tragedies that could have been prevented, or if not entirely prevented, could be greatly reduced.

—Louis Sullivan, M.D.

LESSON ASSIGNMENTS

Review the following assignments in order to schedule your time appropriately. Pay careful attention; the titles and numbers of the textbook chapter, the telecourse guide lesson, and the video program may be different from one another.

Text:

Hales, *An Invitation to Health,*
Chapter 17, "Staying Safe: Preventing Injury, Violence, and Victimization," pp. 568–587 and pp. 592–597.

Video:

"Injury Prevention"
from the series *Living with Health.*

OVERVIEW

We often hear the expression, "It was an accident." In reality, there is no such thing as a true accident. If we begin with the "accident" and work backward, we will always find that if some aspect had happened differently, if a different decision had been made, the outcome would have changed. This concept becomes very important as we look at how injuries most often happen and who is at risk. This lesson also becomes very important when we consider that virtually everyone of us will sustain at least one injury in our life (usually quite a few) and that injuries are the leading cause of death from birth to age forty-five.

Consider the fact that most often your own decision and subsequent action either causes or prevents the incident that leads to injury. If you approach your life with this bit of knowledge, you will be likely to make decisions that reduce your risk for injury. You have heard the expression "driving defensively." Expand this concept to "living defensively."

The other very important part of living a healthy lifestyle is knowing what to do when injury does occur. Each year many lives could be saved and serious injuries prevented if more people knew basic first aid and cardiopulmonary resuscitation (CPR). Many of us have seen the panic that frequently surrounds an emergency situation. Panic inevitably results when people do not know what to do. Spending the short time it takes to learn first aid and CPR makes the difference in knowing what to do. Remember, the life you save may be your own or that of your loved one. A very important part of the decisions we make to achieve a healthy lifestyle include those that will decrease our risk of injury, as well as giving us the knowledge to function effectively if injury does happen.

LEARNING OBJECTIVES

Goal

You should be able to explain reasons injuries happen, types of injuries most frequent in various settings, principles of injury prevention, and basic principles of emergency care.

Objectives

Upon completion of this lesson, you should be able to:

1. Analyze the factors that increase the likelihood of accident or injury, unintentional and intentional, and describe ways that violence can be decreased.

2. List and discuss risks most common in various settings and describe ways to decrease these risks.

KEY TERMS

Look for these items as you proceed through the lesson assignments. Be able to discuss them upon completion of this lesson.

repetitive motion injury (RMI)
computer vision syndrome
heat cramps
heat stress
heat exhaustion
heat stroke
frostnip
frostbite
hypothermia

TEXT FOCUS POINTS

The following focus points are designed to help you get the most from the text. Review them, then read the assignment. You may want to write notes to reinforce what you have learned.

Text: Hales, *An Invitation to Health*, Chapter 17, pp. 568–587 and pp. 592–597.

1. Analyze the factors that increase the likelihood of an accident or injury.
2. Describe the practices of defensive driving that serve to decrease the risk of vehicular accident and injury.
3. What are some of the most common causes of injury at home? How can these be prevented?
4. Explain some of the principles of occupational or on-the-job safety.
5. Discuss common risks encountered in recreational activities and strategies for preventing injury during these activities.
6. What are some of the causes of aggression and violence? How can the incidence of violence be decreased?

VIDEO FOCUS POINTS

The following focus points are designed to help you get the most from the video segment of this lesson. Review them, then watch the video. You may want to write notes to reinforce what you have learned.

Video: "Accidents and Injury Prevention"

1. Discuss the various factors involved in causing accidents and injury. Explain accidents in terms of the agent-host-environment model.
2. Describe safety measures that reduce the risk of injury at home and on the street. Why is taking responsibility for one's own safety so important?
3. Explain the importance of first aid and cardiopulmonary resuscitation in reducing severity of injury.
4. How can individuals reduce their own risk of injury related to violence?

INDIVIDUAL HEALTH PLAN

This portion of the lesson is designed to enable you to use the information you have learned in your own life situation to improve the quality of your life. You should do any exercise assigned, complete the journal portion of the plan, then put this portion of the health plan into practice in your life.

> Complete the Self-Survey, "Are You Doing Enough to Prevent Accidents?" on pages 571–572 in your textbook. Use this as a basis to examine the types of risks in your lifestyle. In your journal, write an evaluation of your greatest risks of injury. Develop a written plan of action to lower your risk of injury. If you have not already learned first aid and CPR, include this in your plan.

RELATED ACTIVITIES

These activities are not required unless your instructor assigns them. They are offered as suggestions to help you learn more about the material presented in this lesson.

1. Interview a paramedic, an emergency care physician, or nurse, and discuss the types of injuries they most often treat and the types of individuals most often involved.

2. Interview a police officer and learn his or her perspective regarding the role violence and alcohol play in injuries.

PRACTICE TEST

After reading the assignment and watching the video, you should be able to answer the Practice Test questions. Tests also include essay questions that are similar to the Text Focus Points and the Video Focus Points. When you have completed the Practice Test questions, turn to the Answer Key to score your answers.

Multiple-Choice

Select the one choice that best answers the question.

1. The leading cause of death in the United States for individuals between the ages of 18-21 is __________.
   A. motor vehicle accidents
   B. suicides
   C. accidental poisoning
   D. fires

2. The best way to avoid getting in a traffic accident is probably __________.
   A. avoiding alcohol while driving
   B. not driving as often in the evening
   C. avoiding freeways and interstates
   D. avoid driving in bad weather

3. All of the following are common accidental injuries at home that you can protect yourself from EXCEPT __________.
   A. poisonings
   B. falls
   C. burns
   D. abuses

4. Good posture and correct positioning of a computer console may help to prevent the development of all of the following injuries EXCEPT __________.
   A. eye strain
   B. repetitive-motion injuries
   C. electro-magnetic field exposures
   D. back strain

5. The heat-related malady which results from prolonged sweating with inadequate fluid replacement is __________.
   A. heat stress
   B. heat stroke
   C. heat exhaustion
   D. heat cramps

6. When the body temperature falls below ninety-five degrees and becomes incapable of warming itself, this is called __________.
   A. hypothermia
   B. hyperthermia
   C. heat exhaustion
   D. cold sweats

7. All of the following are potential causes of aggressive or violent behavior EXCEPT __________.
   A. poverty
   B. substance abuse
   C. mental illness
   D. ethnicity

8. The agent factor in a motorcycle accident is __________.
   A. crowded streets
   B. careless drivers
   C. rainy weather
   D. energy of the motorcycle

9. When riding a motorcycle or a bicycle, it is important to __________.
   A. choose an expensive bike
   B. wear protective gear
   C. use the left lane
   D. avoid freeways

10. An emergency can be defined as __________.
    A. a major accident
    B. a stoppage of breathing
    C. a heart attack
    D. an event the individual cannot handle comfortably

11. A good defense against a perpetrator is to __________.
    A. do the unexpected
    B. carry a firearm
    C. fight the perpetrator
    D. call "help"

Fill-in-the-Blank

Insert the correct word or words in the blank for each item.

12. Doing the same activity over and over again on the job could lead to a condition known as ___________ __________ __________.

13. A life-threatening medical emergency caused by the breakdown of the body's mechanism for cooling itself is heat __________.

14. The blood alcohol level of the driver of a car is considered the ______________ in the agent-host-environment model.

True-False

If the statement is true, write "T" to the left of the statement. If the statement (or any part of the statement) is false, write "F" to the left of the statement.

15. Most houses have adequate safety measures built into them.

16. First aid and cardiopulmonary resuscitation are complicated procedures best left to paramedics and other professionals.

ANSWER KEY

The following provides the answers and references for the Practice Test questions. Focus Points are referenced using the following abbreviations:
T = Text and V = Video

	Answers	Learning Objectives	Focus Points	References
1.	A	1	T1	Hales, p. 570
2.	A	2	T2	Hales, p. 570
3.	D	2	T3	Hales, pp. 576–577
4.	C	2	T4	Hales, p. 578
5.	C	2	T5	Hales, p. 579
6.	A	2	T5	Hales, p. 580
7.	D	1	T6	Hales, p. 583
8.	D	1	V1	Video
9.	B	2	V2	Video
10.	D	2	V3	Video
11.	A	1	V4	Video
12.	repetitive motion injury	2	V4	Hales, p. 578
13.	stroke	2	T5	Hales, p. 579
14.	host	1	V1	Video
15.	F	2	V2	Video
16.	F	2	V3	Video

Lesson 21

Aging

So often when you get to this age, people seem to think you're supposed to run around with people your age and they want to categorize you. . . . There is no reason at all to enjoy people your own age just because they are your own age because age covers the entire spectrum of society.

—Ellen Mallum

LESSON ASSIGNMENTS

Review the following assignments in order to schedule your time appropriately. Pay careful attention; the titles and numbers of the textbook chapter, the telecourse guide lesson, and the video program may be different from one another.

Text:

Hales, *An Invitation to Health*, (Brief edition),
Chapter 14, "Growing Older," reprinted in *Telecourse Guide for Living with Health*, pp. 192–208.

Video:

"Aging"
from the series *Living with Health.*

OVERVIEW

How do you feel about getting older? Really? What is your image of what it is like to age? Intellectually you may be able to accept the idea that we all are aging. Emotionally it may be a different story. If we see being older as being feeble and frail, we may have very strong negative feelings. If we have come to terms with the fact that aging is a normal process that we all share, we will be able to find the "golden" in the golden years.

Though we may think of aging as a time of frailty, nursing home care, and dependency on others, this is the picture of only a few of our aging population. In reality, most older people are living independently and enjoying active, productive lives. Though the older person is at higher risk for certain types of illnesses and injuries, these are by no means inevitable. Much of the quality of our later years is determined by the decisions we make and the lifestyle we live in our earlier years. If we learn to care for our health and develop a healthy, active lifestyle throughout the earlier part of our lives, we are very likely to continue this into our later years, thus improving the quality of our later life.

The concept of aging with dignity is a very important one. If we talk to older people, the thing that means the most to them is maintaining their independence and control over their own destiny—in other words, their dignity. It is important that we keep this in mind as we relate to our aging relatives and friends. We know that good psychosocial support systems and healthy lifestyles are keys to the well-being of the older citizen. The more we help insure that they maintain as much independence as possible, the higher the quality of life they will enjoy.

As we make our own life choices and decisions, we also want to remember how very important these will be to our own chances of aging with dignity and good health. Each of us has significant control over our own destiny—it is up to us to make wise lifestyle choices that will guide us toward the quality of life that we desire.

LEARNING OBJECTIVES

Goal

You should be able to explain the aging process, the impact of issues and lifestyles in the earlier years on the health in the later years, and the problems faced by the elderly.

Objectives

Upon completion of this lesson, you should be able to:

1. Explain the impact aging has on the individual and some of the problems faced by the elderly.

2. Analyze the influence that health issues and lifestyle in the earlier years have on one's well-being in the later years and ways to increase quality of life and life expectancy.

KEY TERMS

Look for these items as you proceed through the lesson assignments. Be able to discuss them upon completion of this lesson.

aging
ageism
gerontologists
hormones
hormone replacement therapy (HRT)
osteoporosis
dementia
Alzheimer's disease

TEXT FOCUS POINTS

The following focus points are designed to help you get the most from the text. Review them, then read the assignment. You may want to write notes to reinforce what you have learned.

Text: *Telecourse Guide for Living with Health*, pp. 192–208 (reprinted from Hales, *An Invitation to Health*, Brief edition).

1. Explain the impact of aging on major body systems and on mental health.

2. Analyze the way in which health issues of the middle years affect health in the later years.

3. Discuss the factors that increase life expectancy or increase the quality of life.

4. List and explain major health and health-related problems faced by older people in our society.

Growing Old

Taken verbatim from: Hales, *An Invitation to Health*, Brief edition

After studying the material in this chapter, you should be able to:

- Explain the impact of aging on major body systems and on mental health.
- List and explain major health-related problems faced by older people in our society.

Although the process of aging is inevitable, you can do a great deal to influence the impact that the passage of time has on you. As a result of the preventive steps you take now, you can expand your "health span"—your years of health and vitality—as well as possibly expand your lifespan. This chapter gives you a preview of the changes age brings, the steps you can take to age healthfully, and ways to make the most of all the years of your life.

Living in a Graying Society

In the last 100 years, the United States and other developed nations have experienced a greater increase in life expectancy than in all of recorded history prior to 1900. Today the elderly account for 13% of the American population.[1] The ranks of the elderly will grow even more in the next few decades, as the 75 million "baby boomers" conceived from 1946 to 1964 pass their sixty-fifth birthdays (Figure 14-1).

Figure 14-1

Tracking the baby-boom generation in the United States.

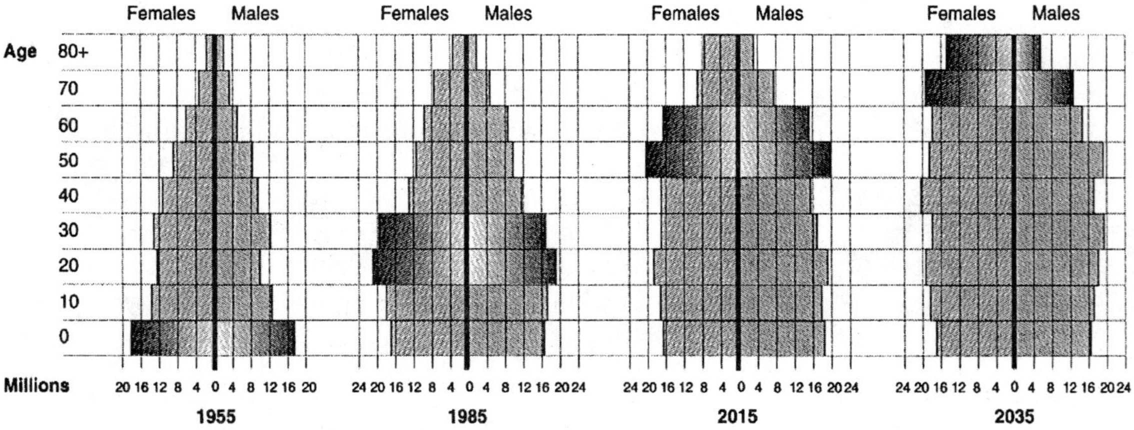

Sources: Population Reference Bureau and U.S. Census Bureau

Regardless of your age, you will be affected by this "graying" of the American population. This is one reason why it's important to bridge the gap in understanding and information between younger and older Americans.

A survey of 1200 men and women by the American Association of Retired Persons (AARP) revealed many misconceptions: 46% of respondents said that most older people could not adapt to change; 65% felt that most older people are lonely; 71% thought that one of every ten elderly Americans lives in an institution (the actual percentage, according to the AARP, is one in twenty).[2] Such negative assumptions may reflect **ageism**, a form of discrimination based on myths about aging and the elderly. As with other forms of discrimination, the best way to confront ageism is to seek accurate information, challenge stereotypes, and get involved in overcoming barriers to understanding.

As Time Goes By

For years, **gerontologists**—specialists in the interdisciplinary field that studies aging—viewed the process of getting older only in terms of deterioration, frailty, the grinding away of time. Today, instead of focusing on the minority of the elderly who go into a steady decline, they are studying the majority of men and women who remain vital and resilient in their later years. The term **optimal aging** refers to the new focus on ways to enhance the well-being and preserve the abilities of older people. Its goal is to enable people to live through old age with the best possible quality of life and the least possible premature disability.

The Impact of Age

From a purely physiological standpoint, the body's finest years come in youth, when lung capacity is greatest, grip is firmest, motor responses are quickest, and physical endurance is longest. After age 30, the body's powers gradually decline. Between the ages of 20 and 80, the percentage of body fat typically increases from 15% to 35% or 40% in men and from 20% to 40% in women. After age 30, the heart's ability to pump blood decreases about 1% each year. At age 30, your heart pumps 3.6 quarts of blood per minute, but at age 70, only 2.6 quarts per minute. Blood pressure rises; circulation slows. These changes simply mean that the average 70-year-old can't compete with a 30-year-old in wrestling or running, but has sufficient energy and stamina for day-to-day functioning (see Figure 14-2).

Figure 14-2: The effects of aging on the body.

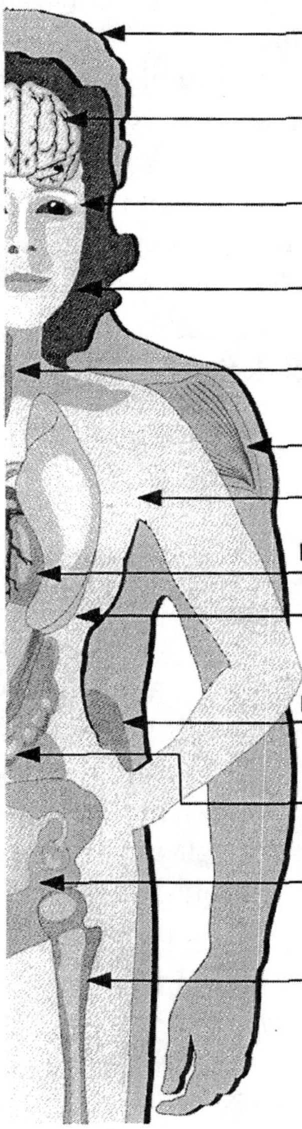

Hair and nails	Hair often turns gray and thins out. Men may go bald. Fingernails can thicken.
Brain	The brain shrinks, but it is not known if that affects mental functions.
The senses	The sensitiviy of hearing, sight, taste, and smell can all decline with age.
Skin	Wrinkles occur as the skin thins and the underlying fat shrinks, and age spots often crop up.
Glands and hormones	Levels of many hormones drop, or the body becomes less responsive to them.
Muscles	Strength usually peaks in the twenties, then declines.
Immune system	The body becomes less able to resist some pathogens.
Heart and blood vessels	Cardiovascular problems become more common.
Lungs	It doesn't just seem harder to climb those stairs; lung capacity drops.
Kidney and urinary tract	The kidneys become less efficient. The bladder can't hold as much, so urination is more frequent.
Digestive system	Digestion slows down as the secretion of digestive enzymes decreases.
Reproductive system	Women go through menopause, and testosterone levels drop for men.
Bones and joints	Wear and tear can lead to arthritic joints, and osteoporosis is common, especially in women.

Aerobic capacity—the amount of oxygen the body can use and the best measure of ability to do work—declines with age. By age 75, a man's aerobic capacity is less than half what it was at age 17; a woman's is about one-third what it was in her twenties. Strength also diminishes slowly. Between the ages of 30 and 70, muscle strength declines about 12% to 15%, and the speed of muscle contraction and coordination drops 25%. Each decade after age 25, men and women lose 3% to 5% of their muscle mass, which often is replaced by fatty tissue. As you get older, bones lose minerals and become softer and shorter. Your muscles weaken and your back slumps. The disks between the bones of the spine also deteriorate, moving those bones closer together. As a result, after 30, both men and women shrink by as much as half an inch in total height with each decade. Basal metabolism—the fundamental chemical process of living—slows down because the aging body requires less upkeep. The rate at which the body turns food into energy declines about 3% every 10 years.[3] As we age, the brain becomes smaller, but mental abilities do not diminish. Aging nerve cells, however, result in slower reaction times and slower movement, and we process information more slowly. A grandfather playing a video game with his 14-year-old grandson will lose every time. However, on tests that involve real-life experience and acquired knowledge, he has the edge.

How Men and Women Age

People of both genders go through numerous physiological changes at midlife. Men experience a decrease in the level of the male sex hormone testosterone, leading to a slowing of the sexual response. Changes in the prostate gland also cause increased urinary urgency, particularly at night (the condition may be alleviated with foods rich in zinc, such as whole grains and milk); the risk of developing prostate cancer grows. For women, the changes at midlife, especially physical ones, can be even more profound. The period from the mid-forties through the mid-sixties is called the climacteric; its most obvious change is the onset of menopause, the end of ovulation and menstruation. An estimated 10% to 15% of women sail through menopause without any significant complaints. At the other end of the spectrum, a similar percentage develop symptoms that make it difficult, if not impossible, for them to function as usual. The majority of women—70% to 80%—are somewhere in between. Most can take advantage of new insight into the processes involved in menopause and new approaches to relieving its symptoms.

The most serious health hazard associated with menopause is an increased risk of heart disease. Throughout a woman's reproductive years, estrogen keeps her arteries supple, prevents blood clots, boosts levels of beneficial high-density lipoproteins (HDL), and decreases harmful low-density lipoproteins (LDL). As estrogen falls at menopause, a woman's heart becomes as vulnerable as a man's. Her HDL slumps; her LDL increases; her risk of blood clots grows; atherosclerotic plaque builds up in her arteries. After age 45, one in nine women has a least one symptom of heart disease. By 65, this figure rises to one in three.

Also at risk are a woman's bones. Although the process of bone loss begins in a woman's thirties, it speeds up to as much at 2% to 5% annually in the first 5 years after menopause. Women with small bones, smokers, and those with a family history of bone problems are at increased risk of fractures and the bone-thinning disease known as osteoporosis, which strikes more than a third of older women (discussed later in this chapter).

Hormone Replacement Therapy (HRT)

Hormone replacement therapy (HRT) is synthetic estrogen, often combined with progesterone, which is given in the form of a pill or a patch to post-menopausal women. It often relieves symptoms of menopause and provides health benefits. The most compelling reason to take replacement hormones is to protect the heart. "Regardless of when a postmenopausal woman starts HRT or for how long she takes it, there is an association with lower incidence of coronary artery disease," says Marianne Legato, M.D., the director of the Partnership for Women's Health at Columbia University. "If a woman has coronary artery disease, HRT may extend her life span by 2½ years. If she doesn't have heart disease, estrogen won't prolong her life, but it will lower her risk of developing cardiovascular problems."[4] HRT also protects a woman's bones. However, the benefits last only as long as the woman takes estrogen, and doctors are still debating whether it's best to start HRT immediately after menopause or later in life.

In addition to these long-term benefits, replacement estrogen relieves hot flashes, improves sleep, alleviates sexual symptoms, makes intercourse more comfortable, and lessens urinary tract problems. Women on HRT report that they think better, remember more, and feel more energetic. They're less prone to many age-related problems, such as tooth loss and driving accidents (possibly a consequence of improved concentration). They also live longer. Compared with women who never used replacement hormones, women who take HRT are less likely to die of what researchers call "all-cause mortality" (that is, for any and every reason). In one analysis of 40,000 postmenopausal women followed for 16 years, the risk of death in those taking estrogen was 37% lower than those who had never taken HRT. The risk of fatal heart disease was 53% lower.[5]

The number-one reason women are wary of HRT is the risk of breast cancer. Although there have been contradictory findings, breast cancer rates generally increase among women who take replacement hormones for prolonged periods. (In various studies, these have extended for 5, 7, or 10 or more years.)[6]

Based on this evidence, physicians may advise against HRT for women who've had breast cancer or who are at high risk for this disease. But for other women, the potential benefits of HRT may outweigh the dangers. Even among those at high risk of breast cancer, the presence of even one risk factor for heart disease tips the balance in favor of HRT.[7] "Women are ten times more likely to die of heart disease than breast cancer," notes Legato. "For many, the risks of not taking HRT are far greater than its use."

Good News about Getting Older

The key to staying vital and healthy in old age is maintaining healthful behaviors throughout life. As many as half of the losses linked to age may be the result not of time's passage but of disuse. "If you don't use it, you lose it," says Dr. James Fries, a Stanford University professor who's done extensive research on aging.

Heredity's Role

Genes aren't destiny, but they have a continuing impact throughout the lifespan. Yet even individuals with genes that contribute to fast aging can modify their impact. What you do to stop the genes that speed up aging is less important than what you do to cooperate with the genes that slow it down. (See Pulsepoints: "Ten Ways to Live Longer.")

Exercise: An Antiaging Pill

Staying in bed for 3 weeks has the same effect on fitness as aging 30 years. At any age, the unexercised body—though free of the symptoms of illness-will rust out long before it could ever wear out. Inactivity can make anyone old before his or her time. Just as inactivity accelerates aging, activity slows it down. The effects of ongoing activity are so profound that gerontologists sometimes refer to exercise as "the closest thing to an antiaging pill." Exercise can reverse many of the changes that occur with age, including increases in body fat and decreases in muscle strength. The bottom line: What you don't do may matter more than what you do.

Pulsepoints: Ten Ways to Live Longer

1. **Exercise regularly**. By improving blood flow, staving off depression, warding off heart disease, and enhancing well-being, regular workouts help keep mind and body in top form.
2. **Don't smoke**. Every cigarette you puff can snuff out 7 minutes of your life, according to the Centers for Disease Control and Prevention.
3. **Watch your weight and blood pressure**. Increases in these vital statistics can increase your risk of hypertension, cardiovascular disease, and other health problems.
4. **Eat more fruits and vegetables**. These foods, rich in vitamins and protective antioxidants, can reduce your risk of cancer and damage from destructive free radicals.
5. **Cut down on fat**. Fatty foods can clog the arteries and contribute to various cancers.
6. **Limit drinking**. Alcohol can undermine physical health and sabotage mental acuity.
7. **Cultivate stimulating interests**. Elderly individuals with complex and interesting lifestyles are most likely to retain sharp minds and memories beyond age 70.
8. **Don't worry; be happy**. At any age, emotional turmoil can undermine well-being. Relaxation techniques, such as meditation, help by reducing stress.
9. **Reach out**. Try to keep in contact with other people of all ages and experiences. Make the effort to invite them to your home or go out with them. On a regular basis, do something to help another person.
10. **Make the most of your time.** Greet each day with a specific goal-to take a walk, write letters, visit a friend.

The Aging Brain

Mental ability does not decline along with physical vigor. Researchers have been able to reverse the supposedly normal intellectual declines of 60-to-80 year olds by tutoring them in problem solving. Reaction time, intellectual speed and efficiency, nonverbal intelligence, and maximum work rate for short periods may diminish by age 75. However, understanding, vocabulary, ability to remember key information, and verbal intelligence remain about the same.

Mental Health

Optimal aging demands a redefinition of who a person is and what makes his or her life worthwhile. Some sources of satisfaction, such as physical challenges or professional achievements, diminish later in life. Yet older people in general feel psychologically better than young people, with fewer worries about themselves and how they look to other people, higher self-esteem, and less loneliness.[8]

The secret of emotional well-being in old age doesn't seem to be professional success or a happy marriage but the ability to cope with life's setbacks without blame or bitterness. In general, psychiatric disorders do not occur more frequently in the elderly. Even depression—which is not uncommon among the elderly—strikes less often in old age than at earlier stages of the life cycle. Those most likely to become depressed often have lost a spouse and have few social supports. The social ties of the elderly are most likely to fray as they retire, move, or lose spouses and close friends.[9]

Intimacy and Sexual Activity

Sexual activity typically decreases in the elderly, but it doesn't end. According to a 1995 national survey by Mark Clements Research, Inc., about 55% of those between ages 65 and 69 remain sexually active. This percentage declines with age—to 48% of those between 70 and 74, 28% of those 75 to 79, 21% of those 80 to 84, and 13% of those over age 85.[10]

Aging does cause some changes in sexual response: Women produce less vaginal lubrication, and it takes longer for an older man to achieve an erection or orgasm and longer to attain another erection after ejaculating. Both men and women experience fewer contractions during orgasm. However, none of these changes reduces sexual pleasure or desire.

Problems of the Elderly

Sadly, life's final decades aren't always golden. Senior citizens may face physical, economic, social, and psychological challenges during what one therapist describes as "the season of loss." They may have to give up many things: gratifying work, cherished friendships, financial and physical independence. Millions are economically vulnerable: a serious illness, the loss of their home in a fire or flood, or other unexpected catastrophes could easily plunge them into poverty. A lack of money limits the options of the elderly and can impair their health. They may not be able to afford nutritious food, regular health checkups, new eyeglasses or hearing aids, or the small pleasures that make life enjoyable. The cumulative impact of such challenges, one often following the other before individuals have a chance to adjust or cope, can take a toll on physical and emotional well-being.

Physical Problems

With the passage of time, many people develop serious diseases such as arthritis, atherosclerosis, and cancer. In the past, elderly men and women often were not treated as aggressively for some conditions, such as cancer, as younger patients. But research has shown that older patients can respond well to aggressive therapeutic approaches and benefit just as much as younger individuals.[11]

Nutritional Needs

Among the elderly, nutritional deficiencies are a serious problem; being underweight can be as great a health risk as being overweight. About 16% of Americans over age 65 consume fewer than 1000 calories a day—too little to provide an adequate supply of vitamins and minerals. Common causes of malnutrition in old age include medications, emotional depression, loss of teeth, swallowing and absorption disorders, lack of money, and difficulties shopping and preparing food. Many nutritionists recommend multivitamin and mineral supplements for the elderly, although they caution against overdosing or taking any single vitamin or mineral without medical supervision.

Osteoporosis

One common problem, especially among elderly women, is osteoporosis, a condition in which losses in bone density become so severe that a bone will break after even slight trauma or injury (see Figure 14-3). Among those who live to age 90, 32% of women and 19% of men will suffer a hip fracture as a result of osteoporosis.[12] Women, who have smaller skeletons, are more vulnerable than men; in extreme cases, their spines may become so fragile that just bending causes severe pain.

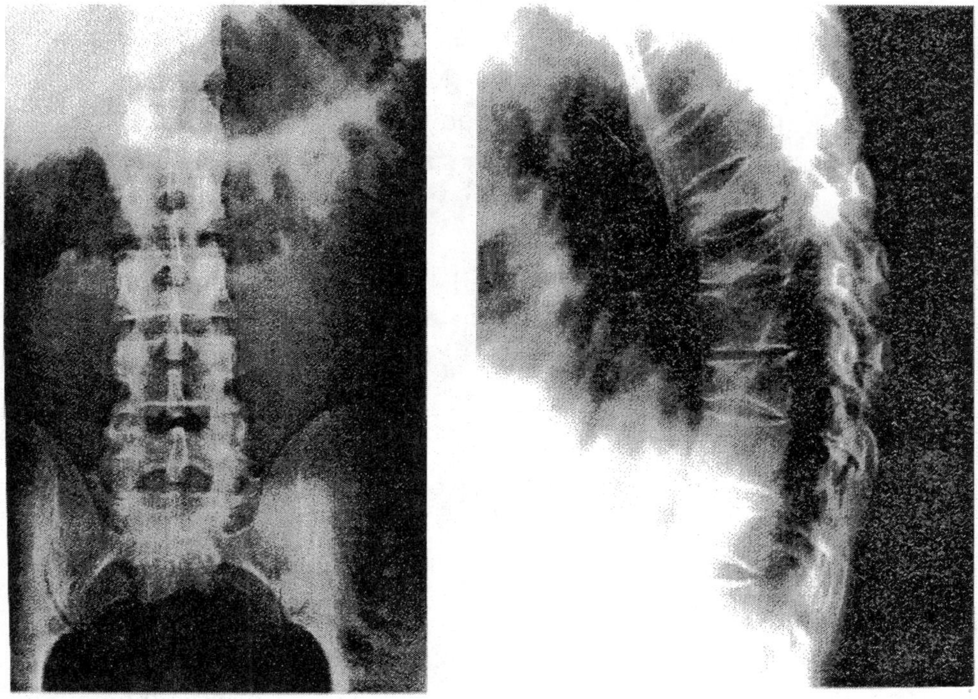

Figure 14-3
Comparison of a normal backbone (left) to one with osteoporosis (right).

Osteoporosis doesn't begin in old age. In fact, the best time for preventive action is early in life. Increased calcium intake, particularly during childhood and the growth spurt of adolescence, can produce a heavier, denser skeleton and reduce the risk of the complications of bone loss later in life. College-age women also can strengthen their bones and reduce their risk of osteoporosis by increasing their calcium intake and physical activity. Adequate dietary calcium in adulthood can help maintain bone density for years.

Various factors can increase a woman's risk of developing osteoporosis, including family history (a mother, grandmother, or sister with osteoporosis, fractures, height loss, or humped shoulders); petite body structure; white or Asian background; menopause before age 40; smoking; heavy alcohol consumption; loss of ovarian function through chemotherapy, radiation, or hysterectomy; low calcium intake; and a sedentary lifestyle.

Substance Misuse and Abuse

Misuse and abuse of prescription and over-the-counter medications occur frequently among the elderly. In part this is because people over age 65 consume one-quarter of all drugs prescribed in the United States. Moreover, many older people have multiple health problems, requiring several medications at the same time. The drugs may interact and cause a confusing array of symptoms and reactions.

Alcohol abuse can be particularly harmful for older men and women because it increases the likelihood of malnutrition, liver disease, heart damage, digestive problems, cognitive impairment, and dementia. Depending on the severity of the problem, older individuals may require close supervision in a hospital during withdrawal.

Psychological Problems

As men and women end their careers, and as friends and loved ones become ill or die, loneliness can become a chronic problem. Women, who generally outlive their husbands, are most likely to find themselves living alone. Whereas seven out of ten men age 75 or older are still married and living with their spouses, seven out of ten women in that age group are widowed. "We have our children and grandchildren and friends," says one woman in her eighties who lives in an apartment complex for elderly widows. "But we do miss our men."

Depression

According to a report by the National Institutes of Health Consensus Development Panel on Depression in Later Life, about 15% of men and women over 65 living in the community experience depression. In nursing homes, the rate is higher: 15% to 25%. Moreover, recurrences are common, with 40% of older persons suffering repeat bouts with depression.[13]

Late-life depression can be particularly hard to spot because older men and women often do not display the typical symptoms, or their symptoms are mistaken for normal signs of aging.[14] Elderly people with physical problems are most prone to depression. Some classic signs of depression—appetite changes, a gain or loss of 5% of body weight in a month, insomnia or excessive sleep, fidgeting or extremely slow movements or speech, fatigue, or loss of energy—may be attributed to medical problems, medications, or old age itself. Depression that develops following an illness or injury, if not identified and treated, can hinder recovery.

The consequences of not recognizing and treating depression late in life can be tragic. Older Americans have the highest suicide rates in our society, with some 8,500 elderly persons killing themselves every year. The suicide rate is five times higher for those aged 65 or older than for younger individuals. And depressed older men and women are also more likely to die of other causes. However, late-life depression can be overcome. With treatment, more than 70% of the depressed elderly improve dramatically.

Mental Deterioration

About 15% of older Americans lose previous mental capabilities, a brain disorder called dementia. Sixty percent of these—a total of 4 million men and women over age 65—suffer from the type of **dementia** called Alzheimer's disease, a progressive deterioration of brain cells and mental capacity.

Women are more likely to develop Alzheimer's than men. By age 85, as many as 28% to 30% of women suffer from Alzheimer's, and women with this form of dementia perform significantly worse than men in various visual, spatial, and memory tests. Estrogen replacement, despite the risks and concerns discussed earlier, may help keep women's brains healthy as they age, particularly for those at high genetic risk for Alzheimer's. In various studies of postmenopausal women, those taking replacement hormones were up to 40% less likely to develop Alzheimer's. And women who do develop Alzheimer's show less mental deterioration if they are taking estrogen.[15]

Often the illness progresses slowly, stealing bits of a person's mind and memory a little at a time. Its victims may withdraw into a world of their own, become quarrelsome or irritable, and say or do inappropriate things. The personalities of individuals with Alzheimer's often change. Some become more stubborn or impulsive; others may become increasingly apathetic, withdrawn, irritable, or suspicious, accusing others of thefts, betrayal, or plotting against them. As cognitive impairment worsens, inhibitions often loosen; they may masturbate or take off their clothes in public. Some become aggressive or violent. Eventually, individuals may forget the names of their close relatives, their own occupations, occasionally even their own names.[16]

Even though no one can restore a brain that is in the process of being destroyed by an organic brain disease like Alzheimer's, medications can control difficult behavioral symptoms and enhance or partially restore cognitive ability. Often physicians find other medical or psychiatric problems, such as depression, in these patients; recognizing and treating these conditions can have a dramatic impact. Most people with Alzheimer's do best in consistent, familiar surroundings, with daily routines, prominently displayed clocks and calendars, nightlights, checklists, and diaries.

Nursing Homes

Many older people need help from another person in performing some daily living activity, such as dressing, walking, bathing, or shopping. In the past, aging parents tended to live with their children's families. That's changed dramatically-not only because children live farther away, or may be separated or divorced, but also because the older parents seem to prefer their independence. Problems can develop, however, when declining health or increasing disability makes it more difficult for the elderly to manage on their own. Home-care services, day care, and foster homes help growing numbers of the elderly by filling the gap between living at home and entering a nursing home.

More than 1.5 million elderly Americans currently live in nursing homes, and their numbers are certain to grow in the coming decades. But such care is expensive and can be substandard, if not abusive. Families of elderly patients mistreated in nursing homes have successfully sued the homes, not for acts that led to death or disability, but for neglect, such as leaving residents in a smelly room or not bathing them or verbal abuse.[17]

Self Survey
What Is Your Aging IQ?

Mark each of the following statements True or False.

1. Everyone becomes senile sooner or later, if he or she lives long enough.
2. American families have by and large abandoned their older members.
3. Depression is a serious problem for older people.
4. The numbers of older people are growing.
5. The vast majority of older people are self-sufficient.
6. Mental confusion is an inevitable, incurable consequence of old age.
7. Intelligence declines with age.
8. "Sex" urges and activity normally cease between ages 55 and 60.
9. If a person has been smoking for thirty or forty years, it does no good to quit.
10. Older people should stop exercising and should rest.
11. As you grow older, you need more vitamins and minerals to stay healthy.
12. Only children need to be concerned about calcium for strong bones and teeth.
13. Extremes of heat and cold can be particularly dangerous to older people.
14. Many older people are hurt in accidents that could have been prevented.
15. More men than women survive to old age.
16. Deaths from stroke and heart disease are declining.
17. Older people on the average take more medications than younger people.
18. Snake-oil salesmen are as common today as they were on the frontier.
19. Personality changes with age, as do hair color and skin texture.
20. Sight declines with age.

ANSWERS

1. False. Even among those who live to be 80 years of age or older, the majority do not develop Alzheimer's disease or forms of brain disease. Senility is a medically meaningless term.
2. False. The American family is still the number one caretaker of older Americans. Most older people live close to their children and see them often; many live with their spouses. Eight out of ten men and six out of ten women live in family settings.
3. True. Depression, loss of self-esteem, loneliness, and anxiety can become more common as older people face retirement, the deaths of relatives and friends, and other such crises often at the same time. Fortunately, depression is treatable.
4. True. By the year 2030, one out of every five people will be over 65 years of age.
5. True. Only 5% of the older population live in nursing homes; the rest are basically healthy and self -sufficient.
6. False. Mental confusion and serious forgetfulness in old age can be caused by Alzheimer's disease or other conditions that cause incurable damage to the brain, but a hundred other problems can cause the same symptoms. A minor head injury, a high

fever, poor nutrition, adverse drug reactions, and depression can all be treated, and the confusion will go away.

7. False. Intelligence per se doesn't decline without reason. Most people maintain or improve their intellect as they grow older.

8. False. Most older people can lead an active, satisfying sex life.

9. False. Stopping smoking at any age reduces the risk of cancer and heart disease and leads to healthier lungs.

10. False. Many older people enjoy, and benefit from, exercises such as walking, swimming, and bicycle riding. Exercise at any age can help strengthen the heart and lungs, and lower blood pressure.

11. False. Although certain requirements, such as that for "sunshine" vitamin D, may increase slightly with age, older people need the same amounts of most vitamins and minerals as do younger people. Older people, in particular, should eat nutritious foods and cut down on sweets, salty snack foods, high-calorie drinks, and alcohol.

12. False. Older people require fewer calories, but adequate intake of calcium for strong bones can become more important as you grow older. This is particularly true for women, whose risk of osteoporosis increases after menopause. Milk and cheese are rich in calcium, as are cooked dried beans, collards, and broccoli. Some people need calcium supplements as well.

13. True. The body's thermostat tends to function less efficiently with age, and the older person's body may be less able to adapt to heat or cold.

14. True. Falls are the most common cause of injuries among the elderly. Good safety practices, including proper lighting and nonskid carpets, can help prevent serious accidents.

15. False. Women tend to outlive men by an average of eight years. There are 150 women for every 100 men over age 65, and nearly 250 women for every 100 men over age 85.

16. True. Fewer men and women are dying of stroke or heart disease. This has been a major factor in the increase in life expectancy.

17. True. The elderly consume 25% of all medications and, as a result, have many more problems with adverse drug reactions.

18. True. Medical quackery is a $10 billion business in the United States. People of all ages are commonly duped into quick cures for aging, arthritis, and cancer.

19. False. Personality doesn't change with age. Therefore, all old people can't be described as rigid and cantankerous. You are what you are for as long as you live. But you can change what you do to help yourself enjoy good health.

20. False. Although changes in vision become more common with age, any dramatic change in vision, regardless of age, may be related to a specific disease.

MAKING CHANGES

Staying Younger Longer

As the above answers indicate, many common beliefs about aging simply aren't true. In fact, you have a great deal of control over how you age; and by changing your health habits, you may be able to buy yourself extra years of life and health. Here are some guidelines that can extend both your "health span"—your active, healthy years—and your lifespan:

- Don't smoke. If you smoke two or more packs of cigarettes a day, you are essentially trading a minute of life for a minute of smoking. You can expect to lose 8.3 years of life you might have lived as a nonsmoker.

- If you drink, don't overdo it. Drinking excessive amounts of alcohol can lead to cirrhosis of the liver, car accidents, pneumonia, high blood pressure, diabetes, and many other life-threatening conditions.

- Eat a low-fat, balanced diet. Some believe a bad diet can decrease the average lifespan six to ten years. Certainly, diet may have a lot to do with your risk of heart disease, colon or breast cancer, and other disorders.

- Watch your weight. Whether or not you're overweight can make a difference in your predisposition to heart attacks, strokes, kidney disease, diabetes, and other disorders.

- Exercise regularly. Exercise may add six to nine years to your life. The fitter you are, the longer you can expect to live.

- Learn to manage stress effectively. Establish a good balance of work and play in your life. Try to keep stress within reasonable limits. Excessive stress can make intense demands on the body and may make some people prone to heart attacks. Learning to manage and control stress effectively can lessen the toll it takes on well-being.

SOURCE: U.S. Department of Health and Human Services, Bethesda, MD: Government Printing Office, 1986.

References

1. Steel, Knight. "Research on Aging: An Agenda for All Nations Individually and Collectively." *Journal of the American Medical Association*, Vol. 278, No. 16, October 22/29, 1997.
2. Stock, Robert. "Senior Class." *New York Times*, June 1, 1995.
3. "Can You Live Longer?" *American Health*, August 1994.
4. Legato, Marianne. Personal interview.
5. Stewart, Donna, and Gail Robinson. *A Clinician's Guide to Menopause.* Washington, DC: Health Press, 1997.
6. "Breast Cancer and Hormone Replacement Therapy: Collaborative Reanalysis of Data from 51 Epidemiological Studies of 52,705 Women with Breast Cancer and 108,411 Women Without Breast Cancer." *Lancet*, Vol. 350, No. 9084, October 11, 1997.
7. LaCroix, Andrea, and Wylie Burke. "Breast Cancer and Hormone Replacement Therapy." *Lancet*, Vol. 350, No. 9084, October 11, 1997.
8. Sheehy, Gail. *New Passages.* New York: Random House, 1995.
9. Hales, Dianne, and Robert Hales. *Caring for the Mind.* New York: Bantam Books, 1995.
10. Mark Clements Research, Inc. "Sex over 65 Survey." August 1995.
11. American Cancer Society. Doll, R., et al. (eds.). *Trends in Cancer Incidence and Mortality.* Plainview, NY : Cold Spring Harbor Laboratory Press, 1994. Skolnick, Andrew. "Leader in War on Cancer Looks Ahead: Talking with Vincent T. DeVita, Jr., M.D." *Journal of the American Medical Association*, Vol. 273, No. 7, February 15, 1995.
12. Krall, Elizabeth, et al. "Bone Mineral Density and Biochemical Markers of Bone Turnover in Healthy Elderly Men and Women." *Journal of Gerontology*, Vol. 52, No. 2, March 1997.
13. Blazer, Dan. "Depression in Late Life." *Health in Mind & Body*, Vol. 2, No. 1, January 1998.
14. Valan, N. M., and D. M. Hilty. "Depression in the Elderly Not Always What It May Seem." *Health in Mind & Body*, Vol. 2, No. 1, January 1998.
15. Gilman, Sid. "Alzheimer's Disease." *Perspectives in Biology & Medicine*, Vol. 40, No. 2, Winter 1997.
16. Lawlor, Brian. *Behavioral Complications in Alzheimer's Disease.* Washington, DC: American Psychiatric Press, 1995.
17. "New Census Report Details Graying of U.S." *HealthSpan*, Vol. 6, No. 1, Summer 1995. Kane, Robert. "Improving the Quality of Long-Term Care." *Journal of the American Medical Association*, Vol. 273, No. 17, May 3, 1995.

VIDEO FOCUS POINTS

The following focus points are designed to help you get the most from the video segment of this lesson. Review them, then watch the video. You may want to write notes to reinforce what you have learned.

Video: "Aging"

1. Describe some of the body changes that occur with aging and the reasons these occur.
2. Explain the psychosocial stages from infancy to old age described by Erikson.
3. What are some of the ways that we can increase the health and quality of our lives as we grow older? Include things that we can do to improve the quality of life for our older relatives and friends.

INDIVIDUAL HEALTH PLAN

This portion of the lesson is designed to enable you to use the information you have learned in your own life situation to improve the quality of your life. You should do any exercise assigned, complete the journal portion of the plan, then put this portion of the health plan into practice in your life.

> Complete the Self-Survey, "What Is Your Aging IQ?" on pages 205–206 in your telecourse guide. What did you learn about your knowledge of the aging process? Now, think about the important older people in your life, the quality of their lives, and your relationships with them. Based on what you have learned in this lesson, how would you evaluate these things? Consider the lifestyle you are leading and the planning (or lack of it) that you are doing for your own later years. In your journal, develop some plans for your life designed to help ensure that you have the opportunity to age with dignity. If there are things that you would like to do differently in your relationships with the important people in your life, include those.

RELATED ACTIVITIES

These activities are not required unless your instructor assigns them. They are offered as suggestions to help you learn more about the material presented in this lesson.

1. Arrange an interview with a gerontologist, geriatric nurse, or other professional who works with senior citizens and discuss the life of senior citizens including their special needs and problems.

2. Visit an older person living in a nursing home and one living independently. Compare their lifestyles, health, feelings, problems, and the quality of their lives.

PRACTICE TEST

After reading the assignment and watching the video, you should be able to answer the Practice Test questions. Tests also include essay questions that are similar to the Text Focus Points and the Video Focus Points. When you have completed the Practice Test questions, turn to the Answer Key to score your answers.

Multiple-Choice

Select the one choice that best answers the question.

1. All of the following are true statements regarding aging in the United States EXCEPT __________.
   A. the most rapidly growing age group of elders in the United States consists of people over the age of 100
   B. the average age of the United States' population is rising
   C. more couples are having children later
   D. today the elderly account for 13 percent of the American population

2. Women are most likely to enter menopause __________.
   A. before age 40
   B. around age 45
   C. after age 50
   D. around age 65

3. Which of the following would seem to be most important to emotional well-being in aging?
   A. Having had a successful career
   B. Coping with life's setbacks without blaming others or being bitter
   C. Having a happy marriage that lasts into old age
   D. Maintaining lifelong friendships and having several hobbies

4. All of the following are potential symptoms of Alzheimer's EXCEPT _______.
   A. aggression
   B. apathy
   C. paranoia
   D. phobias

5. A good alternative to nursing homes for older people who cannot fully manage on their own may be __________.
   A. public hospitalization
   B. medication to boost ability
   C. home-care service
   D. government subsidies

6. The aspect of normal aging over which people have most control is _________.
   A. change of visual acuity
   B. level of fitness
   C. density of bones
   D. elasticity of skin

7. According to Erikson, the period of life when parenting responsibilities decrease and people begin assessing their career achievements is known as __________.
   A. young adulthood
   B. middle age
   C. older adulthood
   D. old age

8. Supports that ensure a higher quality of life in the later years are LEAST likely to include __________.
   A. family and friends
   B. quality of health
   C. specific religious denomination
   D. leisure and pleasure activities

Fill-in-the-Blank

Insert the correct word or words in the blank for each item.

9. Discrimination against an individual based on age is known as __________.

10. The goal of enabling people to live through old age with the best possible quality of life is known as ____________ ____________.

11. The loss of mental capacity with aging is known as ______________.

12. The time when one's children are grown and some outward signs of aging are beginning to occur is termed ______________ _________.

True-False

If the statement is true, write "T" to the left of the statement. If the statement (or any part of the statement) is false, write "F" to the left of the statement.

13. The aging process begins at about age 55.

14. In old age, social relationships, sporting activities, and hobbies are begun as the new focus of life.

15. Lifestyle choices in early life greatly affect health in the later years.

ANSWER KEY

The following provides the answers and references for the Practice Test questions. Focus Points are referenced using the following abbreviations:

T = Text and V = Video

	Answers	Learning Objectives	Focus Points	References
1.	A	1	T1	TG, p. 192
2.	C	2	T2	TG, p. 195
3.	B	2	T3	TG, p. 199
4.	D	1	T4	TG, pp. 203-204
5.	C	1	T4	TG, p. 204
6.	B	1	V1	Video
7.	B	2	V2	Video
8.	C	2	V3	Video
9.	ageism	1	T1	TG, p. 193
10.	optimal aging	2	T2	TG, p. 193
11.	dementia	1	T4	TG, p. 203
12.	middle age	2	V2	Video
13.	F	1	V1	Video
14.	F	2	V2	Video
15.	T	2	V3	Video

Lesson 22

Death and Dying

When I think about what gives me strength to look at dying and not be afraid, I realize that the strength-giving element in my life did not occur two years ago or three years ago; it's not related to the cancer. It's really related to whatever the tenure of my life has been, and it's not changed dramatically, and I'm okay with the fact that I was born, I lived a good life, and I'm dying.

—Mary Stupp

LESSON ASSIGNMENTS

Review the following assignment in order to schedule your time appropriately. Pay careful attention; the titles and numbers of the textbook chapter, the telecourse guide lesson, and the video program may be different from one another.

Text:

Hales, *An Invitation to Health,*
Chapter 18, "When Life Ends," pp. 598–619.

Video:

"Death and Dying"
from the series *Living with Health.*

OVERVIEW

Elisabeth Kübler-Ross called death "the final stage of growth." My friend, Mary, talked of "my last great adventure." Others speak of the "angel of death." What does death mean to you? Have you come to the acceptance of your own mortality? and that of your loved ones? If these questions frighten you or make you uneasy, you are not alone. Many share your fears and uncertainty.

No one really knows what dying is. Many have had similar "near-death" experiences, which have given us a glimpse, but no one actually knows. What we do know is that each of us will experience death, and death is a normal part of the human experience.

The way in which we support dying loved ones and even accept our own mortality depends largely on our own feelings about death and dying. It is important that we understand the process, are able to think about it and to talk about it.

Acceptance of death certainly does not come all at once, and coping with the death of a loved one is not an easy process. Elisabeth Kübler-Ross described stages that one may go through in accepting death. However, she also says that people do not go neatly through these stages, and some never get to the stage of acceptance. Most experts feel that we generally die in much the same manner as we have lived. In other words, if we have led a fairly centered, healthy life, we will be able to accept the idea of death. Our emotional hardiness allows us to cope with the experience of life and death.

All too often our own fears and conflicts make it difficult or impossible to offer support to the very ones we love the most at the time that they need us. Some of us cannot bear to even visit the dying, much less talk of their feelings and thoughts. It is as though if we don't acknowledge death, it will not happen. Dying patients need to talk. They need us to be able to listen and share feelings with them.

An important part of our health is to be able to also accept the concept of dying and death. If we can be at peace with this final stage of growth, our life will be much fuller, much more meaningful.

LEARNING OBJECTIVES

Goal

You should be able to discuss differing views of death, the stages of acceptance of death, the process of dying, and the grieving process.

Objectives

Upon completion of this lesson, you should be able to:

1. Define death, explain the stages of acceptance of death, the factors that affect a person's attitudes about death, and some of the ethical dilemmas surrounding right-to-die issues, including suicide.

2. Discuss some of the issues in the process of dying, the impact of death on grieving survivors, and the grieving process.

KEY TERMS

Look for these items as you proceed through the lesson assignments. Be able to discuss them upon completion of this lesson.

thanatology
coma
persistent vegetative state
advanced directives
do-not-resuscitate (DNR)
living will
holographic will
terminal illness
hospice
near-death experience
autoscopy
transcendence
euthanasia
dyathanasia

TEXT FOCUS POINTS

The following focus points are designed to help you get the most from the text. Review them, then read the assignment. You may want to write notes to reinforce what you have learned.

Text: Hales, *An Invitation to Health*, Chapter 18, pp. 598–619.

1. Define death and explain the stages of emotional acceptance experienced in facing death.

2. Describe some of the ethical controversy surrounding death, the right to die, and the influence of culture on life-and-death decisions.

3. Explain the purposes of advanced directives, including the living will and the holographic will.

4. Describe some of the experiences that the dying patient may encounter in the process of dying. What things are most helpful at this time?

5. Discuss the issues of suicide and euthanasia in the case of terminal illness.

6. List and explain factors affecting the length and intensity of grief. How do the practicalities of funeral planning, and so forth, relate to this?

VIDEO FOCUS POINTS

The following focus points are designed to help you get the most from the video segment of this lesson. Review them, then watch the video. You may want to write notes to reinforce what you have learned.

Video: "Death and Dying"

1. Explain the five stages of acceptance of death described by Elisabeth Kübler-Ross.

2. How can family and friends offer the dying patient emotional support?

3. Why is the grieving process important? Do all people grieve in the same way?

INDIVIDUAL HEALTH PLAN

This portion of the lesson is designed to enable you to use the information you have learned in your own life situation to improve the quality of your life. You should do any exercise assigned, complete the journal portion of the plan, then put this portion of the health plan into practice in your life.

> Complete the Self-Survey, "How Do You Feel About Death?" on pages 603–604 of your textbook. Did any of your answers surprise you or upset you? Think about the feelings you had about death and dying before you started this lesson. In your journal, analyze any feelings that have changed and the way in which they have changed. Describe your current feelings about death and the process of dying. If you find yourself very troubled about death, consider consulting a counselor or clergy member.

RELATED ACTIVITIES

These activities are not required unless your instructor assigns them. They are offered as suggestions to help you learn more about the material presented in this lesson.

1. Contact a hospice facility and discuss hospice care.

2. Talk with health professionals, lawyers, and clergy concerning issues such as organ transplants, living wills, and euthanasia.

3. Visit a funeral home and discuss funeral arrangements with a staff member.

PRACTICE TEST

After reading the assignment and watching the video, you should be able to answer the Practice Test questions. Tests also include essay questions that are similar to the Text Focus Points and the Video Focus Points. When you have completed the Practice Test questions, turn to the Answer Key to score your answers.

Multiple-Choice

Select the one choice that best answers the question.

1. All of the following are forms of death based on physiological occurrences EXCEPT __________.
   A. functional death
   B. cellular death
   C. spiritual death
   D. cardiac death

2. All of the following are stages of reactions individuals experience when facing death EXCEPT __________.
   A. anger
   B. relief
   C. bargaining
   D. depression

3. Which of the following individuals is best responsible for do-not-resuscitate orders on hospital patients?
   A. Family of the patient
   B. Patient's physician
   C. Hospital policy
   D. Combination of all of the above

4. To be terminally ill means that __________.
   A. there is only a slight chance of recovery
   B. there is an endpoint to the illness and it might be death
   C. the patient will die unless some major medical procedure is performed
   D. death is an inevitable occurrence of the disease

5. Which of the following best describes autoscopy?
   A. One sees relatives and loved ones in heaven.
   B. One watches the resuscitation efforts on one's own body from above.
   C. One feels a sense of relief and freedom from pain.
   D. One has a sense of passing into a foreign region.

6. Which of the following best describes transcendence?
   A. One sees relatives and loved ones in heaven.
   B. One watches the resuscitation efforts on one's own body from above.
   C. One feels a sense of relief and freedom from pain.
   D. One has a sense of passing into a foreign region.

7. Voluntary groups that help individuals plan in advance for death are called __________.
   A. hospice workers
   B. memorial societies
   C. funeral homes
   D. crematoriums

8. The impact of death on surviving family members __________.
   A. involves major disruptions, but only briefly
   B. is greatest for those with a lack of social support
   C. is generally more severe for elderly women than for elderly men
   D. is less if the death was more sudden

9. Though the individual may be complaining and relatively talkative, the fourth stage in the acceptance of death includes __________.
   A. anger
   B. bargaining
   C. depression
   D. acceptance

10. In offering support to the dying, confidants should do all the following EXCEPT __________.
    A. appear ready to listen
    B. reassure that things will be fine
    C. talk about death
    D. share feelings of love and acceptance

11. Problems develop when people __________.
    A. express individuality in their grieving
    B. cannot overcome their acute grief
    C. take six months to work through grief
    D. talk frequently about the deceased

Fill-in-the-Blank

Insert the correct word or words in the blank for each item.

12. An individual who is in a total state of unconsciousness is in a _______.

13. The act of allowing someone to commit suicide or helping someone who is terminally ill commit suicide is known as ________________.

14. After individuals recover from the shock and denial of finding that they have a terminal illness, they usually experience ________________.

15. Coming to terms with the death of a loved one usually occurs during the process of ____________.

True-False

If the statement is true, write "T" to the left of the statement. If the statement (or any part of the statement) is false, write "F" to the left of the statement.

16. The depression stage is usually a very quiet one for the dying patient.

17. An important role that friends can play is to listen to whatever the dying patient wants to talk about.

ANSWER KEY

The following provides the answers and references for the Practice Test questions. Focus Points are referenced using the following abbreviations:

T = Text and V = Video

	Answers	Learning Objectives	Focus Points	References
1.	C	1	T1	Hales, p. 600
2.	B	1	T1	Hales, pp. 602, 604
3.	D	2	T3	Hales, p. 605
4.	D	2	T4	Hales, p. 609
5.	B	2	T4	Hales, p. 611
6.	D	2	T4	Hales, p. 611
7.	B	2	T6	Hales, p. 614
8.	B	2	T6	Hales, p. 614
9.	C	1	V1	Video
10.	B	2	V2	Video
11.	B	2	V3	Video
12.	coma	1	T2	Hales, p. 605
13.	euthanasia	1	T5	Hales, p. 612
14.	anger	1	V1	Video
15.	grief	2	V3	Video
16.	F	1	V1	Video
17.	T	2	V2	Video

Lesson 23

Health Self-Care

Each patient carries his own doctor inside him. People have come to us not knowing that truth. We doctors are at our best when we give the doctor who resides in each patient a chance to go to work.

—Albert Schweitzer, M.D.

LESSON ASSIGNMENTS

Review the following assignment in order to schedule your time appropriately. Pay careful attention; the titles and numbers of the textbook chapter, the telecourse guide lesson, and the video program may be different from one another.

Text:

Hales, *An Invitation to Health*,
Chapter 10, "Consumerism, Complementary/Alternative Medicine, and the Health Care System," pp. 332–338, p. 347, and pp. 360–363.
"Hales Health Almanac," pp. A1–A36.

Video:

"Health Self-Care"
from the series *Living with Health.*

OVERVIEW

Earlier in the history of this country, people took a great deal of responsibility for their own health care. The main reasons for this were their isolation from doctors and unavailable transportation. Then people began to rely heavily on the more accessible physicians and their newer "wonder" drugs. Now people are again realizing that they can care for many of their own minor illnesses. They have also developed more interest in some of the alternative health-care methods. In a time when our health-care delivery systems are overcrowded and very expensive, it is a wise person who uses good judgment in knowing when professional health care is needed and when caring for one's own minor illness is possible.

The Internet has also brought a whole new group of health issues. How do we evaluate online health information? What sites are accurate and of high quality? We have to be wise "surfers" in order to take full advantage of this wealth of material called the "web."

The health-activated person has adopted a lifestyle that minimizes risk of illness and injury. However, we all know that even a healthy person sometimes falls prey to a "bug" or minor injury. As we learn to listen to our body when it gives us clues that all is not well, and how to determine how serious our condition may be, we will be able to make healthy decisions about how to care for ourselves when the balance is disturbed.

Most minor illnesses are self-limiting and do not require prescription drugs. Often a simple relief of the symptoms is all the body needs to heal itself. In fact it is good to remember the old saying, "If you ignore a cold, it goes away in a week, if you treat it, it goes away in seven days." A healthy body has a remarkable amount of resiliency and ability to heal itself, if allowed. Usually all that's needed is the simplest self-care. If the symptoms don't go away, if they worsen, or if more serious signs are present, it is time to get professional care. If you have doubts, call your physician's office or consult your college health center.

Through all of this, remember: we have been talking about a healthy body. Once again we are reminded that we are responsible for the lifestyle that insures that our health is optimal. We can't delegate this responsibility to anyone else, not even our physician.

LEARNING OBJECTIVES

Goal

You should be able to explain the importance of being health conscious and of good self-care, medical tests, some components of the home medicine chest, and the first steps to be taken in an emergency.

Objectives

Upon completion of this lesson, you should be able to:

1. Discuss the importance of self-care, how to evaluate online medical advice, and some appropriate self-care actions for dental health and other aspects of one's health.

2. Identify some of the most common symptoms of illness and the medical tests most often performed.

KEY TERMS

Look for these items as you proceed through the lesson assignments. Be able to discuss them upon completion of this lesson.

vital signs
gum disease
plaque
gingivitis
periodontitis
flap surgery
medical history

TEXT FOCUS POINTS

The following focus points are designed to help you get the most from the text. Review them, then read the assignment. You may want to write notes to reinforce what you have learned.

Text: Hales, *An Invitation to Health*, Chapter 10, pp. 332–338, p. 347, and pp. 360–363. "Hales Health Almanac," pp. A1–A36.

1. Define self-care and describe appropriate self-care actions for various conditions. How do you evaluate online medical advice?

2. Describe the important actions needed to maintain good dental health.

3. Explain the value of the home medicine chest, some items to be included in it and the first steps to be taken in an emergency.

4. Identify some of the most common symptoms of illness and the medical tests most often performed, and explain what the results of medical tests could indicate.

VIDEO FOCUS POINTS

The following focus points are designed to help you get the most from the video segment of this lesson. Review them, then watch the video. You may want to write notes to reinforce what you have learned.

Video: "Health Self-Care"

1. Describe some of the problems that an individual can treat without seeking professional medical care. Include the signs and symptoms that indicate that professional care is needed.
2. What are the behaviors that indicate that a person is health-activated or proactive in maintaining good health?
3. Under what circumstances are over-the-counter medications useful? How does one choose a medication for a particular problem?
4. What are some of the important goals and concerns for the health of the people of the United States in the future?

INDIVIDUAL HEALTH PLAN

This portion of the lesson is designed to enable you to use the information you have learned in your own life situation to improve the quality of your life. You should do any exercise assigned, complete the journal portion of the plan, then put this portion of the health plan into practice in your life.

> Complete the Self-Survey, "Are You a Savvy Health-Care Consumer?" on page 347 of your textbook. Did you know the correct answers to these questions? In your journal, list the characteristics about yourself that you consider to be health-conscious or non-health-conscious in the way you make decisions about issues. Based on this, develop a written plan for yourself that will help you become more health-conscious.

RELATED ACTIVITIES

These activities are not required unless your instructor assigns them. They are offered as suggestions to help you learn more about the material presented in this lesson.

1. Take an inventory of the over-the-counter (OTC) drugs in your home. Check the expiration dates and discard any that are out of date. Do the same for any prescription drugs you have.

2. In a visit to your pharmacy, read the labels of several OTC drugs meant for the same condition. Do you find similarities? Differences? Note the number of ingredients and the cost of each.

3. As you see advertisements for health-care products, do you see signs of quackery, misrepresentation, or "stretching the truth"?

PRACTICE TEST

After reading the assignment and watching the video, you should be able to answer the Practice Test questions. Tests also include essay questions that are similar to the Text Focus Points and the Video Focus Points. When you have completed the Practice Test questions, turn to the Answer Key to score your answers.

Multiple-Choice

Select the one choice that best answers the question.

1. Which of the actions listed below are needed for individuals to help keep medical costs down while insuring quality?
   A. Learn how to spot medical problems.
   B. Know what to expect from health-care professionals.
   C. Know where to turn for appropriate treatment.
   D. All of the above are necessary.

2. Normal respiration rate for an adult is __________.
   A. 10-15 breaths per minute
   B. 25-30 breaths per minute
   C. 20-25 breaths per minute
   D. 15-20 breaths per minute

3. Children of today have far less tooth decay because of ___________.
   A. good luck
   B. fluoridated water and toothpaste
   C. better toothbrushes
   D. better brushing techniques

4. The most serious form of gum disease is ___________.
   A. gingivitis
   B. plaque
   C. periodontitis
   D. otitis

5. The following are actions that should be taken if broken bones are suspected EXCEPT ___________.
   A. straighten out the fracture
   B. keep the person warm and calm
   C. do not try to push a broken bone back if it is sticking through the skin
   D. splint unstable fractures

6. The individual usually does NOT need to see a physician for ___________.
   A. abdominal pains
   B. common colds
   C. temperatures of 104° F
   D. earaches

7. Behaviors that indicate a person is health-activated and being proactive in health include all the following EXCEPT ___________.
   A. exercising regularly
   B. eating a healthy diet
   C. refraining from seeing a physician except for emergencies
   D. doing self-assessments of one's health

8. Over-the-counter medications are useful to __________ .
   A. alleviate symptoms of minor ailments
   B. eliminate infections
   C. prevent colds and flu
   D. cure many diseases

9. Goals for improving the health of the people of the United States include all the following EXCEPT __________ .
   A. decreasing violence
   B. strengthening the family
   C. increasing dependence on physicians
   D. improving nutrition

Fill-in-the-Blank

Insert the correct word or words in the blank for each item.

10. In a healthy adult at rest, the normal heart rate is approximately ____ beats per minute.

11. The early stage of gum disease is known as ______________.

12. The first aid action of artificially providing oxygen to an individual who has no heartbeat is CPR or ____________________ ____________________.

13. A person who is proactive and takes responsibility for individual health is termed ______________________.

True-False

If the statement is true, write "T" to the left of the statement. If the statement (or any part of the statement) is false, write "F" to the left of the statement.

14. It is usually safe for individuals to treat their colds and minor wounds by themselves.

15. In spite of advertising claims, many over-the-counter medications have similar ingredients.

ANSWER KEY

The following provides the answers and references for the Practice Test questions. Focus Points are referenced using the following abbreviations:
T = Text and V = Video

	Answers	Learning Objectives	Focus Points	References
1.	D	1	T1	Hales, p. 334
2.	D	1	T1	Hales, p. 335
3.	B	1	T2	Hales, p. 345
4.	C	1	T2	Hales, p. 345
5.	A	2	T3	Hales, p. A20
6.	B	1	V1	Video
7.	C	1	V2	Video
8.	A	2	V3	Video
9.	C	1	V4	Video
10.	72	1	T1	Hales, p. 335
11.	gingivitis	1	T2	Hales, p. 345
12.	cardiopulmonary resuscitation	2	T3	Hales, p. A22
13.	health-activated	1	V2	Video
14.	T	1	V1	Video
15.	T	2	V3	Video

Lesson 24

Health-Care Delivery Systems

The practice of medicine in its broadest sense includes the whole relationship of the physician with his patient. Good practice presupposes an understanding of modern medicine, but it is obvious that sound professional training should include a much broader equipment.

—Dr. Francis Peabody, *JAMA*, 1927
(Journal of the American Medical Association)

LESSON ASSIGNMENTS

Review the following assignments in order to schedule your time appropriately. Pay careful attention; the titles and numbers of the textbook chapter, the telecourse guide lesson, and the video program may be different from one another.

Text:

Hales, *An Invitation to Health*,
Chapter 10, "Consumerism, Complementary/Alternative Medicine, and the Health Care System," pp. 339–363.

Video:

"Health-Care Delivery Systems"
from the series *Living with Health.*

OVERVIEW

If there is any question about our interest and concern about health-care delivery systems, just read a newspaper, listen to a television newscast, look on the Internet, or listen to a political speech. The whole country seems preoccupied with the large issue of health care. Unfortunately, we frequently don't understand the relationships that we as individuals have with this huge issue. We ask ourselves:

"How do we fit in? What should we do? What can we really do?" Though we may feel there are no answers to all this, there really are some things that we as individuals can do.

Clearly, the most important thing that we can do is make lifestyle decisions that insure that we keep ourselves as healthy as possible. Second, we can educate ourselves so that we are wise patients who take an active role in our recovery if we become ill. We should carefully choose our health-care providers so that we work with them as a team to maintain our health. We should be clear and reasonable about our health needs and expectations and intelligently evaluate the care we receive. We must not be passive consumers of health care who give up our rights when we enter the health-care delivery system. Third, we must do what we can to help control the costs of health care. This involves using all the things we have learned to be health-activated and health-conscious.

If each of us, from the single individual to the largest institution, truly becomes involved in doing our part, the health-care delivery system and problems in this country will surely "take a turn for the better."

LEARNING OBJECTIVES

Goal

You should be able to describe different types of health-care providers and facilities; identify factors in selecting, assessing, dealing with, and evaluating providers and facilities; analyze the major issues facing the United States health-care delivery system; and explain alternative forms of therapy.

Objectives

Upon completion of this lesson, you should be able to:

1. Describe the types of health-care professionals, their selection and assessment, the doctor-patient relationship, and alternative medical models.

2. Discuss the various types of health-care facilities, the issues facing the United States health-care delivery system, and ways health care is evaluated.

KEY TERMS

Look for these items as you proceed through the lesson assignments. Be able to discuss them upon completion of this lesson.

Pap smear
false positive
false negative
negligence
over-the-counter (OTC)
informed consent
malpractice
quackery
complementary and alternative medicine (CAM)
holistic
integrative medicine
chiropractic
herbal medicine
mind-body medicine
acupuncture
ayurveda
biofeedback
homeopathy
naturopathy
visualization
primary care
diagnostic-related group (DRG)
home health care
managed care
indemnity
health maintenance organization (HMO)
preferred provider organization (PPO)

TEXT FOCUS POINTS

The following focus points are designed to help you get the most from the text. Review them, then read the assignment. You may want to write notes to reinforce what you have learned.

Text: Hales, *An Invitation to Health*, Chapter 10, pp. 339–363.

1. Describe the different types of health-care professional. Identify and discuss factors in selecting and assessing a health-care professional.

2. List the different types of health-care facilities. What role does each play in the health-care system? What are some of the issues to consider in assessing and dealing with health-care institutions?

3. Discuss the doctor-patient relationship. Why is the annual physical examination important? Include a discussion of patient's rights.

4. Analyze the issues facing the United States health-care delivery system today. Include the issues of managed care and insurance of health care.

5. Explain the importance of medical research and the ways health care is evaluated. How can online medical advice be evaluated?

6. Describe some of the complementary/alternative forms of medicine and what research has shown about its effectiveness.

VIDEO FOCUS POINTS

The following focus points are designed to help you get the most from the video segment of this lesson. Review them, then watch the video. You may want to write notes to reinforce what you have learned.

Video: "Health-Care Delivery Systems"

1. Why is it so important to be an informed patient and to be actively involved in one's own health care?

2. Describe some guidelines that should be used when choosing and evaluating a health-care provider.

3. What are the important factors in maintaining good communications between patient and physician? Include a discussion of the patient's rights.

INDIVIDUAL HEALTH PLAN

This portion of the lesson is designed to enable you to use the information you have learned in your own life situation to improve the quality of your life. You should do any exercise assigned, complete the journal portion of the plan, then put this portion of the health plan into practice in your life.

> In your journal, list your own resources for health care: physician, dentist, clinic, hospital insurance, etc. Describe the ways you utilize these services. Are you health-conscious? If there are ways in which you could improve, develop a plan for doing this.

RELATED ACTIVITIES

These activities are not required unless your instructor assigns them. They are offered as suggestions to help you learn more about the material presented in this lesson.

1. Compare and contrast health insurance plans, coverage, and cost of several different companies. Include Medicare and Medicaid. What were your findings?

2. Interview some physicians, dentists, and acquaintances of yours and find out their expectations of the health professional/patient relationship.

PRACTICE TEST

After reading the assignment and watching the video, you should be able to answer the Practice Test questions. Tests also include essay questions that are similar to the Text Focus Points and the Video Focus Points. When you have completed the Practice Test questions, turn to the Answer Key to score your answers.

Multiple-Choice

Select the one choice that best answers the question.

1. Which of the following physicians do more than half of women choose as a primary physician?
   A. Obstetrician
   B. Pediatrician
   C. Internist
   D. Psychiatrist

2. Which of the following is probably the best strategy to take when selecting a new physician for your care?
   A. Make a decision on a doctor and stick with it.
   B. Do not ask too many questions because most doctors don't like this.
   C. Ask about the physician's philosophy of treatment care.
   D. All of the above are good strategies.

3. All of the following are fundamental principles of acupuncture EXCEPT _____.
   A. a cycle of energy circulating through the body controls health
   B. pain is a result of a disturbance in energy flow
   C. needles are inserted at meridians
   D. massage forms a basis for treatment

4. A Veterans Administration hospital is an example of __________.
   A. a community facility
   B. a private facility
   C. a public facility
   D. a teaching facility

5. The primary drawback to managed care as a means of health-care delivery is that __________.
   A. a third party makes decisions on what is acceptable care for a patient
   B. the cost is becoming prohibitively high in relation to care received
   C. too many unnecessary tests are being performed
   D. physicians have little incentive to use these systems

6. A second opinion is usually NOT needed when the __________.
   A. individual and physician agree about treatment
   B. need for major surgery is indicated
   C. individual questions the treatment
   D. diagnosis is unclear

7. Steps in choosing a physician do NOT include __________.
   A. checking with the local medical society
   B. interviewing several physicians
   C. looking in the yellow pages of the phone book
   D. considering the environment in the office

8. The most important aspect in making an accurate diagnosis is the __________.
   A. electrocardiogram
   B. patient's history
   C. blood tests
   D. physical exam

Fill-in-the-Blank

Insert the correct word or words in the blank for each item.

9. The medical test done to screen for the presence of cervical cancer is known as a _______ ________.

10. The newer form of health-care system in the United States that relies on a third party to determine the necessity of medical treatment is known as ___________ ________.

True-False

If the statement is true, write "T" to the left of the statement. If the statement (or any part of the statement) is false, write "F" to the left of the statement.

11. The patient who takes an active role in treatment usually has a better outcome.

12. The general office environment is of little importance in the choice of a physician.

13. If either the physician or the patient questions the diagnosis or treatment plan, a second opinion should be sought.

14. Though many rights are maintained, the right to privacy must be given up when seeking medical treatment.

ANSWER KEY

The following provides the answers and references for the practice test questions. Focus points are referenced using the following abbreviations:

T = Text and V = Video

	Answers	Learning Objectives	Focus Points	References
1.	A	1	T1	Hales, p. 339
2.	C	1	T3	Hales, p. 339
3.	D	1	T6	Hales, p. 354
4.	C	2	T2	Hales, p. 356
5.	A	2	T4	Hales, p. 358
6.	A	1	V1	Video
7.	C	1	V2	Video
8.	B	1	V3	Video
9.	Pap smear	1	T3	Hales, p. 342
10.	managed care	2	T4	Hales, p. 358
11.	T	1	V1	Video
12.	F	1	V2	Video
13.	T	1	V3	Video
14.	F	1	V3	Video

Lesson 25

Environmental Health

The whole point is we're on a road now that is leading to extinction. What we're doing now to the planet and the ways we do it are not sustainable. . . . If we remember that our health and the health of the planet are synonymous, inseparable, then we'll start behaving differently toward the planet because we want health.

—Hal Flanders

LESSON ASSIGNMENTS

Review the following assignments in order to schedule your time appropriately. Pay careful attention; the titles and numbers of the textbook chapter, the telecourse guide lesson, and the video program may be different from one another.

Text:

Hales, *An Invitation to Health*,
Chapter 19, "Working Toward a Healthy Environment," pp. 620–639.

Video:

"Environmental Health"
from the series *Living with Health.*

OVERVIEW

The technological revolution of the twentieth century has at one time been a boon and a curse to the planet and its people. On the one hand, it brought advances and wonders beyond belief. On the other, it seemed to be dooming the planet to an early death.

As we consider the relationship of the environment and our health, we must realize that these two are inextricably intertwined. The health of the planet is our health and our health is the health of the planet. Each affects the other in more ways than we might imagine. All of the issues of advancing technology and their environmental impact are trade-offs. We cannot nor should we do without the health benefits that technology offers us. However, we cannot ignore the fact that the health of our planet is deteriorating rapidly and having damaging effects on our health. We cannot continue to use up our natural resources and pollute our air and water as though these are infinite. They are finite, and when they are depleted or polluted beyond use, we will become extinct as other species of the earth already have. Of all the dilemmas facing us in this twenty-first century, this is perhaps the most critical to our future. We can no longer hang on to the belief that technology will solve these problems. We must act individually to solve the simpler problems and then cooperatively develop solutions to the complex ones if our planet and its peoples are to survive and thrive.

LEARNING OBJECTIVES

Goal

You should be able to discuss the cyclical nature of the impact of the environment on the individual's health and the impact of the individual on the health of the environment, the extent to which pollution affects the health of the population, various environmental health problems, and the important actions necessary to help solve these.

Objectives

Upon completion of this lesson, you should be able to:

1. Explain the major hazards to the survival of the planet and some of the actions individuals can take to protect the environment.

2. Discuss the issues of air, noise, water, chemical, and other types of pollution which include radiation.

KEY TERMS

Look for these items as you proceed through the lesson assignments. Be able to discuss them upon completion of this lesson.

ecosystem
multiple chemical sensitivity (MCS)
zero population growth (ZPG)
pollution
pollutant
mutation
mutagen
teratogen
fuels
greenhouse effect
ozone layer
precycling
recycling
smog
acid rain
decibels (db)
hertz
endocrine disruptors
chlorinated hydrocarbons
organic phosphates
dioxins
polychlorinated biphenyls (PCBs)
electromagnetic fields (EMFs)
video display terminal (VDT)
microwaves
ionizing radiation
irradiation

TEXT FOCUS POINTS

The following focus points are designed to help you get the most from the text. Review them, then read the assignment. You may want to write notes to reinforce what you have learned.

Text: Hales, *An Invitation to Health*, Chapter 19, pp. 620–639.

1. List and explain the major hazards to the survival of the planet.

2. Discuss some actions individuals can take to protect the environment.

3. Describe the issues related to air pollution, both outdoor and indoor. What can be done to make the air cleaner and decrease the risk of exposure to indoor pollutants?

4. Explain the problems of noise pollution.

5. Analyze the issues related to water and water supply.

6. Discuss the problems of chemical and other types of pollution.

7. What are some of the risks associated with the various forms of radiation? How does the individual protect against these?

VIDEO FOCUS POINTS

The following focus points are designed to help you get the most from the video segment of this lesson. Review them, then watch the video. You may want to write notes to reinforce what you have learned.

Video: "Environmental Health"

1. Explain the cyclical process of the impact that individuals have on the environment and the environment has on the individual.

2. Why is it important to be involved in individual and cooperative action to protect the health of the environment and, in turn, our own health?

3. What are some of the things that individuals can do every day to improve the health of the environment and themselves?

INDIVIDUAL HEALTH PLAN

This portion of the lesson is designed to enable you to use the information you have learned in your own life situation to improve the quality of your life. You should do any exercise assigned, complete the journal portion of the plan, then put this portion of the health plan into practice in your life.

> Complete the Self-Survey, "Are You Doing Your Part for the Planet?" on page 627 of your textbook. In your journal, note the things that you need to change and the things you do well. On the basis of this, develop a plan for improvement.

RELATED ACTIVITIES

These activities are not required unless your instructor assigns them. They are offered as suggestions to help you learn more about the material presented in this lesson.

1. Interview local representatives of private and government environmental protection agencies and find out what major environmental problems exist in your area, what is being done to improve these, and what role you might play in the solution.

PRACTICE TEST

After reading the assignment and watching the video, you should be able to answer the Practice Test questions. Tests also include essay questions that are similar to the Text Focus Points and the Video Focus Points. When you have completed the Practice Test questions, turn to the Answer Key to score your answers.

Multiple-Choice

Select the one choice that best answers the question.

1. The shrinking of the protective ozone layer above the earth has led to an increase in the incidence of __________.
   A. breast cancer
   B. skin cancer
   C. heart disease
   D. respiratory disease

2. Which of the following woods is a rainforest wood?
   A. Ash
   B. Mahogany
   C. Walnut
   D. Cherry

3. In which city would you be most likely to find gray air or sulfur-dioxide based smog?
   A. Chicago
   B. Los Angeles
   C. San Francisco
   D. Denver

4. The unit of measurement used to determine the intensity of sound is known as a __________.
   A. decibel
   B. hertz
   C. rad
   D. PCB

5. Which of the following is the reason for the high rate of chlorine in American drinking water?
   A. The high number of swimming pools in the United States results in contamination of water.
   B. It is added to the drinking supply to kill bacteria.
   C. Chlorine is a naturally occurring agent in most groundwater.
   D. Animal wastes contain chlorine which gets in lakes and streams.

6. All of the following are potential symptoms of pesticide poisoning EXCEPT __________.
   A. constipation
   B. vomiting
   C. mental confusion
   D. respiratory distress

7. The greatest percentage of exposure people have to ionizing radiation in the United States is from __________.
   A. medical X-rays
   B. nuclear power plants
   C. building supplies used in the home
   D. natural sources

8. The relationship of humans to the other species on the planet can be described as __________.
   A. advanced
   B. separate
   C. interrelated
   D. independent

9. Solving environmental health problems does NOT include more __________.
   A. political policy
   B. individual action
   C. cooperative efforts
   D. technological development

10. A sign of the air quality in an area is the __________.
    A. velocity of the wind
    B. growth of lichens
    C. amount of acid rain
    D. density of the trees

Fill-in-the-Blank

Insert the correct word or words in the blank for each item.

11. A combination of smoke, gases, and fog in a mixture of industrial and commercial pollutants is known as ________.

12. The relationship between the health of the individual and the health of the environment is ____________________.

True-False

If the statement is true, write "T" to the left of the statement. If the statement (or any part of the statement) is false, write "F" to the left of the statement.

13. The relationship between the health of the environment and the health of the individual is a cyclical one.

14. A key to solving community environmental problems is through cooperative action.

15. There are few areas in the United States that have very low amounts of air pollution.

16. Eating higher on the food chain, with more processed and prepackaged foods, will increase individual health and the health of the environment.

ANSWER KEY

The following provides the answers and references for the Practice Test questions. Focus Points are referenced using the following abbreviations:

T = Text and V = Video

	Answers	Learning Objectives	Focus Points	References
1.	B	1	T1	Hales, p. 622
2.	B	1	T2	Hales, p. 628
3.	A	2	T3	Hales, p. 628
4.	A	2	T4	Hales, p. 630
5.	B	2	T5	Hales, p. 633
6.	A	2	T6	Hales, pp. 633–634
7.	D	2	T7	Hales, p. 635
8.	C	1	V1	Video
9.	D	1	V2	Video
10.	B	1	V2	Video
11.	smog	2	T3	Hales, p. 627
12.	cyclical or interrelated	1	V1	Video
13.	T	1	V1	Video
14.	T	1	V2	Video
15.	T	1	V2	Video
16.	F	1	V3	Video

Lesson 26

A Celebration of Health

I truly believe that every human being consists of a physical, an emotional, an intellectual, and a spiritual quadrant . . . which work together in total harmony and wholeness . . . only if we have learned to accept our physicalness, if we love and accept our natural emotions without being handicapped by them, without being belittled when we cry, when we express natural anger, when we are jealous in order to emulate someone else's talents, gifts, or behavior. Then we will be able to understand that we have only two natural fears, one of falling and one of loud noises. All other fears have been given to us by grown-ups who projected their own fears onto us, and have passed them from generation to generation.

Most important of all, we must learn to love and to be loved unconditionally. Most of us have been raised as prostitutes. I will love you 'if.' And this word 'if' has ruined and destroyed more lives than anything else on this planet earth. It prostitutes us, it makes us feel we can buy love with good behavior or good grades. We will never develop a sense of self-love and self-reward. If we were not able to accommodate the grown-ups, we were punished, rather than being taught by consistent loving discipline. As our teachers taught, if you had been raised with unconditional love and discipline, you will never be afraid of the windstorms of life. You would have no fear, no guilt, and no anxieties, the only enemies of men. Should you shield the canyon from the windstorms, you would never see the beauty of their carvings.

—Elisabeth Kübler-Ross, M.D., *On Life After Death*

LESSON ASSIGNMENTS

Review the following assignments in order to schedule your time appropriately. Pay careful attention; the titles and numbers of the textbook chapter, the telecourse guide lesson, and the video program may be different from one another.

Text:

Hales, *An Invitation to Health*,
Review Chapter 1, and others that you feel you need.

Video:

"A Celebration of Health"
from the series *Living with Health.*

OVERVIEW

We have shared a long journey, you and I, over the miles, through lives, experiences, and learning. Soon we will part, each to continue our own life. Before we part, think back to the beginning. Remember we talked about the dimensions of health: physical, emotional, intellectual, environmental, social, and spiritual. How many times have we seen these in people's lives? How many times have we heard them talk of these? Even more important we have talked about our lifestyle decisions and choices that either increase the quality of our health or detract from it. As you think back, think of all the different people you have met, some very like yourself, some very different. If you saw yourself in some of the people and situations, was it with celebration or was it with pain?

We have a few more people to meet before we part. All the people you have met have been special in their own way. The people you will now meet you may or may not recognize. Each has made lifestyle decisions to expand one of the dimensions of their health beyond that which most of us achieve. Each started a personal journey to health in much the same way as you and I, but somewhere along the way, they made some incredible decisions in their own lifestyles. Their lives now are, as yours and mine are, a reflection of these decisions and their outcomes. As you meet them, think of your own life and health. What decisions have you made? What lifestyle choices and decisions will you make? Your future and your health are up to you. My hope is that the future will find you **living with health**!

LEARNING OBJECTIVES

Goal

You should be able to apply the concept of health in the dimensions—physical, emotional, intellectual, social, environmental, and spiritual—to your own life and describe aspects of your own lifestyle that support your health and well-being in the dimensions.

Objectives

Upon completion of this lesson, you should be able to:

1. Explain the aspects of your own lifestyle that improve the physical dimension of your health.
2. Discuss the aspects of your own lifestyle that develop the emotional/psychological dimension of your health.
3. Analyze the aspects of your own lifestyle that expand the intellectual dimension of your health.
4. Discuss the aspects of your own lifestyle that sustain the social dimension of your health.
5. Describe the aspects of your own lifestyle that deepen the spiritual dimension of your health.
6. Explain the aspects of your own lifestyle that support the environmental dimension of your health.

KEY TERMS

There are no new terms in this lesson.

TEXT AND VIDEO FOCUS POINTS

The following questions are designed to help you get the most from the textbook review assignment and the video segment of this lesson. Review them before you watch the video. After reviewing the textbook chapters and viewing the video segment, write responses to reinforce what you have learned.

1. What are the changes in your own physical health lifestyle that support your health? Examine diet, exercise, rest, alcohol, drug and medication use, tobacco use, and other aspects that impact physical health. What are your future plans and goals?

2. How have you grown in your emotional/psychological health lifestyle choices? Examine your self-concept, self-esteem, coping abilities, relationships with others, stress management activities, alcohol and drug use, and other aspects that influence emotional health. What do you plan for the future?

3. How have you increased lifestyle behaviors in the intellectual dimension? Examine your study habits; learning activities; working patterns; choices in books, movies, and television; and any other activities that support your intellectual growth. What goals and plans do you have for the future?

4. What lifestyle decisions have you made to enhance the social dimension of your health? Examine leisure time activities, relationships with family and friends, community volunteer activities, and other aspects that influence the social portion of your well-being. What plans have you made for the future?

5. How do your behaviors, beliefs, and values support the spiritual dimension of your life? Examine the relationship of your behavior with your beliefs and values, your respect for others, valuing of the environment, and other aspects that develop the spiritual dimensions.

6. What actions do you take to support the environmental dimension of your health? Examine such things as recycling, product usage, littering, and other actions that impact the environment. How do you value the environment and the planet Earth?

INDIVIDUAL HEALTH PLAN

This portion of the lesson is designed to enable you to use the information you have learned in your own life situation to improve the quality of your life. You should do any exercise assigned, complete the journal portion of the plan, then put this portion of the health plan into practice in your life.

> After reviewing your health, lifestyle status, and goals at the beginning and throughout the course, write in your journal an evaluation of the present status of your health and lifestyle. Has your health changed or improved in any way? What progress have you made toward goals you have set? Have you changed any of your goals and plans? Update your lifestyle plan for the immediate future and for your long-term health goals.

RELATED ACTIVITIES

These activities are not required unless your instructor assigns them. They are offered as suggestions to help you learn more about the material presented in this lesson.

1. Select someone you know that you think exemplifies a lifestyle that is well-balanced among the dimensions. Talk with that person and find out what lifestyle choices, decisions, and even trade-offs have been necessary to achieve this balance.

PRACTICE TEST

There are no new objective test items in this lesson. Your Individual Health Plan serves as your review essay questions.

Contributors

We gratefully acknowledge the valuable contributions to this course from the following individuals. The titles were accurate when the video programs were recorded, but may have changed since the original taping.

LESSON 1— "INVITATION TO HEALTH"

Steven N. Blair, P.E.D., Director of Epidemiology, Cooper Institute for Aerobics Research, Dallas, Texas

LESSON 2—"STRESS"

James W. Pennebaker, Ph.D., Professor of Psychology, Southern Methodist University, Dallas, Texas

LESSON 3—"EMOTIONAL HEALTH"

Pedro M. Perez, M.D., Medical Director, Children and Adolescent Services, Green Oaks Hospital, Dallas, Texas

Alvin F. Poussaint, M.D., Senior Associate of Psychiatry, Judge Baker Children's Center, Boston, Massachusetts

LESSON 4—"INTELLECTUAL WELL-BEING"

W. Robert Beavers, M.D., Clinical Professor of Psychiatry, University of Texas Southwestern Medical Center, Dallas, Texas

LESSON 5—"FITNESS AND EXERCISE"

Steven N. Blair, P.E.D., Director of Epidemiology, Cooper Institute for Aerobics Research, Dallas, Texas

Peter G. Snell, Ph.D., Assistant Professor of Medicine and Physiology, University of Texas Southwestern Medical Center, Dallas, Texas

LESSON 6—"DIET AND NUTRITION"

Arlyn Hackett, Chef, Director of Chef Arlyn Hackett's Kitchen, A Cooking School Host, PBS series *Health Smart Gourmet Cooking,* San Diego, California

LESSON 7—"WEIGHT MANAGEMENT"

Toni Beck, M.A., Tom Landry Sports Medicine and Research Center, Dallas, Texas

Joseph H. McVoy, Jr., Ph.D., Director, Association for the Health Enrichment of Large People; Director, Eating Disorders Program, Saint Alban's Psychiatric Hospital, Radford, Virginia

Peter D. Wood, D.Sc., Ph.D., Professor of Medicine and Associate Director, Stanford Center for Research in Disease Prevention, Stanford University, Palo Alto, California

LESSON 8—"INTIMATE RELATIONSHIPS"

Robert A. Johnson, International Lecturer and Author

Toby Myers, Ed.D., Director, The PIVOT Project of Aid to Victims of Domestic Abuse; Lifetime Board Member, Texas Council on Family Violence, Houston, Texas

LESSON 9—"SEXUALITY"

Barbara S. Cambridge, Ph.D., Associate Professor of Obstetrics and Gynecology, University of Texas Southwestern Medical Center, Dallas, Texas

Sue James, M.S., Clinical Supervisor, Dallas County Rape Crisis and Child Sexual Abuse Center, Dallas, Texas

LESSON 10—"REPRODUCTION AND SEXUAL HEALTH"

Carin Hanratty, R.N., P.N.P., Pediatric Coordinator for Drug Exposed Babies, Parkland Memorial Hospital, Dallas, Texas

Timothy R.B. Johnson, M.D., Professor and Chair, Obstetrics and Gynecology, University of Michigan Health System, Ann Arbor, Michigan

LESSON 11—"PARENTING"

Alvin F. Poussaint, M.D., Senior Associate of Psychiatry, Judge Baker Children's Center, Boston, Massachusetts

John R. Shepperd, Investigator, Criminal District Attorney's Office, Dallas County, Texas

LESSON 12—"COMMUNICABLE DISEASES"

John G. Bartlett, M.D., Chairman, Department of Infectious Diseases, The Johns Hopkins University School of Medicine, Baltimore, Maryland

Ted L. Brown, M.S., Environmental Specialist, New Mexico Environmental Department, Santa Fe, New Mexico

Charles P. Felton, M.D., Chief, Division of Pulmonary Medicine, The Harlem Hospital Center, New York City, New York

Pam Reynolds, M.S., Environmental Specialist, New Mexico Environmental Department, Santa Fe, New Mexico

LESSON 13—"AIDS AND SEXUALLY TRANSMITTED DISEASES"

Elisabeth Kübler-Ross, M.D., President, Elisabeth Kübler-Ross Center, Head Waters, Virginia

Jonathan M. Mann, M.D., M.P.H., Francois Xavier Bagnoud Professor of Health and Human Rights, Harvard School of Public Health, Boston, Massachusetts

L. Laurie Scott, M.D., Fellow, Maternal-Fetal Medicine, University of Texas Southwestern Medical Center, Dallas, Texas

LESSON 14—"CARDIOVASCULAR DISEASE"

Pamela S. Douglas, M.D., Director, Non-Invasive Cardiology, Beth Israel Hospital, Boston, Massachusetts; Associate Professor of Medicine, Harvard Medical School, Boston, Massachusetts

Richard Soltes, M.D., Internal Medicine, Dallas Diagnostic Association, Dallas, Texas

LESSON 15—"TREATMENT AND PREVENTION OF CARDIOVASCULAR DISEASE"

Reginald L. Washington, M.D., Vice President, Rocky Mountain Pediatric Cardiology, P.C., Denver, Colorado

LESSON 16—"CANCER"

James W. Bowen, Ph.D., Vice President for Academic Affairs, Professor of Virology, University of Texas M.D. Anderson Cancer Center, Houston, Texas

Judy A. Gerner, Director, Anderson Network, University of Texas M.D. Anderson Cancer Center, Houston, Texas

Bernard Levin, M.D., Vice President for Cancer Prevention (ad interim), Chairman, Department of Gastrointestinal Medical Oncology and Digestive Diseases, University of Texas M.D. Anderson Cancer Center, Houston, Texas

S. Eva Singletary, M.D., Associate Professor of Surgical Oncology, The University of Texas M.D. Anderson Cancer Center, Houston, Texas

LESSON 17—"DRUGS"

Cheryé C. Callegan, M.D., Chief, Substance Abuse Services, Timberlawn Psychiatric Hospital, Dallas, Texas

J. Pat Evans, M.D., Medical Director, Tom Landry Sports Medicine and Research Center, Dallas, Texas

Thomas R. Kosten, M.D., Associate Professor of Psychiatry, Yale University School of Medicine, New Haven, Connecticut

LESSON 18—"ALCOHOL"

Robin A. LaDue, Ph.D., Clinical Psychologist, Fetal Alcohol and Drug Unit, University of Washington Medical School, Seattle, Washington

LESSON 19—"TOBACCO"

Jacqueline C. Flowers, M.P.H., M.Ed., Board of Directors, American Lung Association, New York City, New York

Gary Harris, M.D., Professor and Interim Chair, Department of Medicine, The University of Texas Health Science Center, San Antonio, Texas

LESSON 20—"INJURY PREVENTION"

Richard A. Newbrey, Lieutenant, Medical Services Officer, Medic One Program, Seattle Fire Department, Seattle, Washington

Richard A. Schieber, M.D., Medical Epidemiologist, Centers for Disease Control and Prevention, Atlanta, Georgia

Hal L. Spiegel, CTRS, Program Specialist SCI Team, Baylor Institute for Rehabilitation, Dallas, Texas

Gary R. Strand, Chief, Medic One Program, Seattle Fire Department, Seattle, Washington

Louis W. Sullivan, M.D., President, Morehouse School of Medicine; Former Secretary, U.S. Department of Health and Human Services, Atlanta, Georgia

LESSON 21—"AGING"

William J. Evans, Ph.D., Chief, Human Physiology Laboratory, USDA Human Nutrition Research Center on Aging, Tufts University, Boston, Massachusetts

Charles S. Wolfe, M.A., Ed.S., Consultant and Lecturer, Charles S. Wolfe and Associates, Inc., Aventura, Florida

LESSON 22—"DEATH AND DYING"

Elisabeth Kübler-Ross, M.D., President, Elisabeth Kübler-Ross Center, Head Waters, Virginia

LESSON 23—"HEALTH SELF-CARE"

Marvin Greenberg, RPh., Owner and Pharmacist in Charge, Greenberg's Drugs, Dallas, Texas

Elizabeth H. Gremore, R.N., M.S., C.H.E.S., Health Education Coordinator, McKinley Health Center, University of Illinois at Urbana-Champaign, Urbana, Illinois

Albert G. Mulley, Jr., M.D., M.P.P., Chief, General Internal Medicine, Massachusetts General Hospital, Boston, Massachusetts

Louis W. Sullivan, M.D., President, Morehouse School of Medicine; Former Secretary, U.S. Department of Health and Human Services, Atlanta, Georgia,

LESSON 24—"HEALTH-CARE DELIVERY SYSTEMS"

Mary Ellen Hernandez Bluntzer, M.D., Internal Medicine, Family Systems Medicine, Dallas, Texas

LESSON 25—"ENVIRONMENTAL HEALTH"

Andres E. Garcia-Rivera, M.S., Director, Environmental Health, Cornell University, Ithaca, New York
Amy Martin, Environmental Science Writer, Dallas, Texas

LESSON 26—"A CELEBRATION OF HEALTH"

Liz Carpenter, Author, Lecturer, and Journalist, Austin, Texas
Sara Hickman, Musician, Artist, and Humanitarian, Dallas, Texas
Barbara Jordan, LL.D., Lyndon B. Johnson Centennial Chair in National Policy, The Lyndon B. Johnson School of Public Affairs, University of Texas, Austin, Texas
Julian D. Pinkham, M.S., M.S.W., Member, Yakima Indian nation, Toppenish, Washington
Peter G. Snell, Ph.D., Olympic Gold Medalist - 800 m - 1960, Olympic Gold Medalist - 800 m - 1964, Olympic Gold Medalist – 1,500 m – 1964; Assistant Professor of Medicine and Physiology, University of Texas Southwestern Medical Center, Dallas, Texas